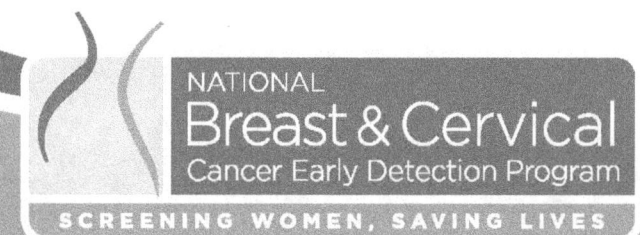

NATIONAL Breast & Cervical
Cancer Early Detection Program
SCREENING WOMEN, SAVING LIVES

Engaging | Building | Expanding

AN NBCCEDP PARTNERSHIP DEVELOPMENT TOOLKIT

MARCH 2011

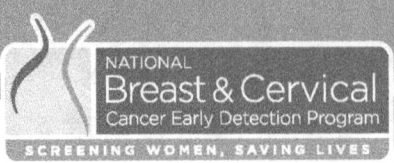

NATIONAL Breast & Cervical
Cancer Early Detection Program
SCREENING WOMEN, SAVING LIVES

Dear Colleagues:

As I reflect on the past 20 years of the Centers for Disease Control and Prevention's (CDC) National Breast and Cervical Cancer Early Detection Program (NBCCEDP), I applaud the efforts of the programs and individuals that are dedicated to saving women's lives through education and early detection. Together, since 1991, you have served more than 3.7 million women in-need who otherwise may not have received these vital education and screening services.

Partners—on both the local and national level—have been critical to our successes over the years. Partners play a key role in helping programs meet their goals through funding, in-kind support, complementary activities to recruit priority populations or educate women, or other expertise. To assist you in building upon these successes, we have created, "Engaging, Building, Expanding: An NBCCEDP Partnership Development Toolkit." The toolkit equips your program with resources to identify, engage, and secure new partners or expand existing partnerships.

The development of the toolkit was informed by research with a number of NBCCEDP programs. A needs assessment and in-depth interviews with program directors helped identify what materials would be most helpful to programs in developing partnerships. To ensure that the materials developed met program needs, we tested materials and messages with program directors and CDC program consultants. We also engaged NBCCEDP's national partners throughout the process.

In this changing health care environment, there are numerous opportunities for programs to develop new partnerships to meet the challenges of the future. It is an important time to communicate your program's public health screening expertise and accomplishments to stakeholders and current partners as well as potential new partners.

The NBCCEDP's public health model effectively reaches and assures quality screening services for low-income, disadvantaged women. Programs and partners can be critical allies in collaborating to increase quality screening through activities such as these:

- Support or provide patient navigation and case management
- Develop and disseminate public information and education programs
- Improve the education, training, and skills of health professionals
- Monitor the quality of screening procedures
- Evaluate effectiveness through appropriate surveillance or program-monitoring activities

I encourage you to use this toolkit to identify potential new partners, and strengthen and sustain collaborations with current partner organizations.

I look forward to continuing our work together and hearing about your future accomplishments.

Sincerely,

Faye L. Wong, M.P.H.
Branch Chief, Program Services Branch
CDC Division of Cancer Prevention and Control

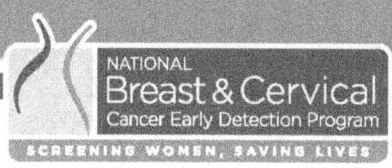

Introduction

Engaging, Building, Expanding: An NBCCEDP Partnership Development Toolkit

Recognizing that National Breast and Cervical Cancer Early Detection Program (NBCCEDP) grant recipients have varying levels of partnership experience, this toolkit has something for everyone. For programs with little partner experience, the toolkit provides how-to's and basic information on starting partnerships or conducting public relations activities. For those with robust partner experience, there are fact sheet templates, new partner ideas, and other branding tools to boost your current partnership efforts. Use the elements of the toolkit that are most applicable to your program's skills and needs.

Toolkit Contents

In addition to providing new resources for partnership development, the toolkit consolidates and highlights previously received partnership trainings, presentations, and similar materials in one easy-to-reference location. Items in the toolkit were created to serve different purposes and audiences; some items are for distribution to women or partners, while others are for internal use to help build your program's partnership skills. The contents are grouped into three categories:

- *Partnership Development Resources:* to help build upon your program's skills for partnership development with how-to's and sample outreach materials.
- *Materials for Distribution by Programs:* to help you make your case with external audiences, such as existing and potential partners or women.
- *Branding Tools:* to help highlight your program's affiliation to the national program through co-branding.

The list below describes the purpose and intended audience of each item in the toolkit.

Partnership Development Resources

Partnership Development Guide—provides overview of partnerships and step-by-step guide for initiating and maintaining them.

Introduction to Public and Media Relations—reviews the importance of public relations and outlines how to approach various tactics, including media relations. Contains instructions for conducting media relations, including how to develop relationships with the media and how to write a press release.

Talking Points—provides key messages about NBCCEDP, the importance of breast and cervical cancer screening, the need for partnerships, and the benefits of partnerships. Can be adapted for individualized partner outreach.

Making Your Case—outlines steps for approaching potential partners, including how to prepare, what to emphasize when reaching out to partners, and how to follow up to maintain the relationship.

Ways to Work With Partners—outlines ways to work with partners, including potential assets and ways to collaborate. Detailed case studies of successful partnerships are included online.

Working with Our National Partners—summarizes best ways to work with NBCCEDP's national partners: American Cancer Society, Avon Foundation for Women, and Susan G. Komen for the Cure.®

Sample Elevator Speech—provides sample language to be used in 30-second introduction to your program and the benefits of partnering.

Sample Pitch Letter—provides sample language to be used in letters to potential partner organizations.

Sample Answers to Common Partner Questions—provides sample language to answer common questions from partners about the need for and benefits of partnerships.

Introduction

Resources—lists online resources from government sites related to public education, statistics and data, and program planning. Including relevant CDC education materials and campaigns.

Materials for Distribution by Programs[1]

About the Program—provides key background information about NBCCEDP, including goals, target audiences, and achievements to date. Can be used with potential partners to emphasize the association with the national program. Programs can insert their contact information and logo. Includes versions featuring photos of American Indian and Hispanic women.

Breast Cancer Facts—explains breast cancer risk, symptoms, and screening recommendations in plain language. Can be used with potential partners and women. Programs can insert their contact information and logo. Includes versions featuring photos of African American, American Indian, Asian American, and Hispanic women.

Cervical Cancer Facts—explains cervical cancer risk, symptoms, and screening recommendations in plain language. Can be used with potential partners and women. Programs can insert their contact information and logo. Includes versions featuring photos of African American, American Indian, Asian American, and Hispanic women.

Why You Should Partner with NBCCEDP Programs—explains why programs need partners, outlines the benefits of partnerships, and gives examples of partner activities. A handout to share with potential partners. Programs can insert their contact information and logo. Includes a version featuring photos of American Indian women.

Program Profile Template—customizable profile listing key program information, including number of women served. Programs can insert their own data and other information. Can be used with potential and existing partners.

Thank You Letter and Recognition Certificate—acknowledge partner support. Programs can insert their contact information and logo. Can be used with existing partners.

Technical Instructions for Customizing Materials—provides technical guidance and specifications on how to add program information and logos to partnership development materials.

Branding Tools

NBCCEDP Brand Identities and Affiliation Badges—Refreshed brand identity, 20th anniversary brand identity, and affiliation badges that programs can use to denote affiliation with the national program. Usage Terms and Conditions are also provided to outline guidelines for use.

PowerPoint Template—designed template that can be used for presentations to partners. Programs can insert their contact information and logo.

Word Document Template—designed template that can be used for communications with partners. Programs can insert their contact information and logo.

Where to Find the Toolkit

The toolkit is available on CD and for download on the NBCCEDP Resource site (www.nbccedp.org). Visit the site for additional materials and updates. If you have any questions about the toolkit, please contact CDC's Division of Cancer Prevention and Control, Program Services Branch at 770-488-4880.

Notes

1 The fact sheets contain similar content to previously available materials. An updated design reflects the new NBCCEDP brand, providing a suite of materials to share with potential partners.

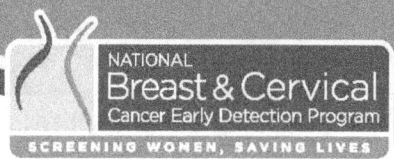

Partnership Development Guide

A partnership can be a relationship between as few as two parties, or it can involve a larger number of individuals and organizations (e.g., a network, coalition, or consortium). The basic assumption of a partnership is that when individuals or organizations join together, they will be more successful in their collective efforts than they could be as individual players—making the best use of different but complementary resources. To be most successful, partnerships should have a clear purpose, add value to the work of the partners, and be carefully cultivated and evaluated. The strongest partnerships occur when both mutual and individual goals are served.

Partnerships help programs of the National Breast and Cervical Cancer Early Detection Program (NBCCEDP) reach their goals by:

- Expanding and maximizing resources
- Coordinating program activities
- Overcoming obstacles to the recruitment of priority populations
- Promoting the delivery, improvement, and evaluation of breast and cervical cancer services

While there is no single formula to create a perfect partnership, this guide outlines key components for successful partnership development: determining needs, assessing potential partners, developing the partnership, and maintaining and sustaining a partnership. It also lists specific steps you can take to build lasting relationships. This document focuses on building and maintaining one-on-one relationships rather than groups or coalitions, but many of these principles can be implemented for groups as well.

A partnership can provide:

- Additional skills and expertise (e.g., planning, design, and implementation of community assessments or program evaluation; provision of training and technical assistance; development and distribution of educational materials)
- Increased understanding of, and access to, priority populations for enhanced outreach and public education
- Increased opportunities for promotion
- Coordination of public education about the issues related to breast and cervical cancer
- Advice on key medical and community issues (e.g., participation on medical advisory board, community advisory groups; assistance with guideline development)
- Increased access to data and interpretation of data
- Links to diagnostic services, treatment, survivorship counseling, and care
- Support for shaping policy change
- Individualized support for patients (e.g., transportation, translation)
- Additional venues through which quality screening can be provided
- Staffing, facilities, or amenities for meetings

For more ideas, including success stories, refer to *Ways to Work With Partners* in this toolkit.

Partnership Development Guide

Determining the Need for Partnerships

A partnership should be initiated to meet specific strategic needs. Assessing the current situation by asking key questions will help you determine your program's needs:

- Where are we having difficulties reaching our goals and objectives (e.g., reaching priority populations, enlisting providers, conducting community assessments, accessing and interpreting other data, evaluating the effectiveness of outreach efforts)?
- How will a partnership benefit our program as a whole (e.g., extending the reach of our message, providing additional funds, providing access to specific skill sets)?
- What are some critical activities that must be sustained, expanded, or improved?
- What program activities could be done more effectively with a strategic partner?
- How might a strategic partnership assist in program efforts?
- What are the benefits of a partnership, and are there any costs to consider? (See Table 1 below.)

Continue to assess your program's needs on a regular basis to determine how you can best collaborate with partners to accomplish your goals.

Assessing Potential Partners

Finding the right partner is critical. Programs should consider the following:

- Which partner could help our program better achieve its goals and objectives?
- What potential partners have been identified?
- What is the expected outcome of the partnership?
- Have we sought out new and nontraditional partners (e.g., organizations serving priority populations, such as lesbians, women with disabilities, and women from racial and ethnic minority communities)?
- Do we have a history of good relations with the potential partner?
- What specific resources will this potential partner contribute to the outcomes or products expected from the partnership?
- What might be some potential drawbacks in partnering with this organization?
- What resources would be valuable? Who has those resources?
- Could collaboration reduce costs or make reallocating funds possible?
- Does the organization understand and support our priorities or have similar priorities?
- Is there a person (a champion) who will work to make sure the partnership happens?

TABLE 1. COST-BENEFIT ANALYSIS FOR NBCCEDP PROGRAMS

POTENTIAL BENEFITS	POTENTIAL COSTS
Increased networking	Time expenditure of scarce resources
Increased information sharing	Loss of autonomy in shared decision making
Access to resources	Lack of direction in the partnership, leading to frustration
Access to the priority population	Perceived lack of appreciation or recognition
Attainment of the desired outcomes from the partnership's efforts	Burnout
Personal recognition and enhanced skills	Lack of necessary skills
	Perceived pressure for additional commitment

Engaging, Building, Expanding: An NBCCEDP Partnership Development Toolkit
Partnership Development Resources: Partnership Development Guide

March 2011

2

Partnership Development Guide

A program also should consider:

- **Benefits or entitlements to offer the partner.** Possibilities include increased visibility, increased access to priority populations, increased networking opportunities, staff development, technical assistance, connections to key stakeholders, improved image, and a high return on investment.

- **Shared goals.** In a reciprocal partnership, there is both a common goal that is advanced by partners working together and individualized benefits for each partner.

There are many different types of organizations that NBCCEDP programs can consider for a partnership. You may want to focus your efforts on the categories of partners below. See *Ways to Work With Partners* in this toolkit for ideas on how to work with these types of partners.

- **Corporations:** National businesses with local branches, local businesses in the community, or major employers

- **Local Government Entities:** Cancer registries, NCI's Cancer Information Service, CDC's Comprehensive Cancer Control Program, federal agencies' offices of women's health, state and local public health agencies/initiatives, state and local offices for aging or minority health, Indian Health Services, Medicare, or elected officials

- **Community-based Organizations:** Cultural groups, civic organizations, health organizations focused on priority audiences, local charitable nonprofits, community leaders, community and migrant health centers

- **Faith-based Organizations:** Churches, synagogues, mosques, or other places of worship, as well as nonprofit organizations with religious affiliations

- **NBCCEDP's National Partners:** American Cancer Society, Avon Foundation for Women, Susan G. Komen for the Cure®

- **Cancer Groups:** Local chapters of national cancer-focused organizations, or local cancer-focused nonprofits

- **Cancer Alliances and Coalitions**

- **Medical Service Providers:** Hospitals, private practice providers, clinics, nonprofit providers, professional organizations whose members are health care providers, or managed care organizations

- **Universities**

Steps for Developing a Partnership

The following steps are offered as suggestions for initiating a partnership. However, each program will need to assess its own situation to determine which steps will be most useful.

1 Research the potential organization, its assets, and the benefits of partnership to determine the appropriate level of partnership between the program and the potential partner. There are various levels of partnership activities, from exchanging information to sharing resources, including:

- **Networking**—exchanging information for mutual benefit

- **Coordinating**—altering activities for mutual benefit to achieve a common purpose

- **Cooperating**—sharing resources (e.g., staff, financial, technical) to achieve a common purpose for mutual benefit

- **Collaborating**—enhancing each other's capacity for mutual benefit and a common purpose

Engaging, Building, Expanding: An NBCCEDP Partnership Development Toolkit
Partnership Development Resources: Partnership Development Guide

March 2011

3

Partnership Development Guide

2 Determine the available resources the program can contribute to the partnership. Shared resources can include a variety of human, financial, and technical contributions, including program or community knowledge, staffing, stakeholder time, physical property, and access to people and/or funding.

3 Develop a document that outlines the mutual benefits of partnership.

4 Know your program and be able to describe it in a succinct manner. You should be able to answer: What does your program do? Why does it matter? How has your program been successful previously? Partners want to associate with programs that can articulate their challenges and successes. Review the *Sample Elevator Speech* and *Making Your Case* in this toolkit for examples.

5 Meet with the potential partner in person, if possible. Because a critical component of a partnership is relationship building, in-person meetings are preferable.

6 Take the time to establish rapport and build trust. Building a strong relationship takes time.

7 Give a general overview of the program (if the potential partner is unfamiliar with NBCCEDP). Use *About the Program* in this toolkit.

8 Explain the program's specific needs and why the partnership would be helpful. The *Talking Points* in this toolkit may be a helpful starting point.

9 Ask about the potential partner's organization and perspective, keeping in mind findings from background research.

10 Learn about the culture of this potential partner—that is, the values, beliefs, etc., that should be taken into consideration when working together. In addition to your own research, this information can be gleaned by observing communication styles, asking direct questions, listening carefully, and asking others who have worked with this partner in the past. Based on your research, adapt your outreach and communications to "speak their language," fit their style and preferences, and ensure it is relevant to their organization.

11 Ask what needs the partner has, and discuss how the program might help meet those needs. Bring ideas from your preparatory research.

12 Ask what resources the partner can contribute to the partnership. Examples of resources include a variety of human, financial, and technical contributions, including program or community knowledge, staffing, stakeholder time, physical property, and access to people and/or funding. Be prepared with specific ideas from your initial research.

13 Make a clear and specific "ask" of the partner. If possible, your "ask" should be task-oriented with a beginning and an end. Don't expect partners to know what is needed; make it as easy for them as possible to partner with you.

Formalizing the Partnership

Once an organization has agreed to partner with your program, it is important to formalize the relationship. One way is to develop a partnership action plan, which could outline a shared vision or mission statement and agreed-upon objectives for the partnership. Defining roles and responsibilities is also important; when appropriate, develop timelines, clarify with your partner who is in charge of each task, and identify a contact person for regular communication.

The partnership action plan might also include:

- Agreed-upon decision-making procedures (e.g., who will decide what and how).
- Ground rules for effective ways of working together
- Anticipated problems or "rough spots," and identified strategies for addressing them
- Additional resources needed to accomplish the goals that are mutually agreed on

Some organizations may be more comfortable formalizing the partnership through a memorandum of understanding (MOU), contract, or some other written document. If you or your partner would prefer this, consult your program's legal department for advice on exact wording.

Engaging, Building, Expanding: An NBCCEDP Partnership Development Toolkit
Partnership Development Resources: Partnership Development Guide

March 2011

4

Partnership Development Guide

Before you engage in partnership activities, discuss together how you define success, and agree upon how to measure or evaluate the partnership's success. This might include periodic documentation or paperwork (e.g., progress reports).

Maintaining and Sustaining a Partnership

A professional partnership takes time, nurturing, and respect. The following suggestions will help you work more effectively with a partner:

- Communicate regularly. Agree on a mutually convenient time and method for "checking in," either verbally or through email.

- Develop a feedback plan for assessing how the partnership is working for both parties. Build on successes, address problems, and explore ways to enhance the partnership.

- Respect the partner's boundaries, structure, procedures, and processes.

- Express appreciation through verbal or written comments.

- With their permission, give your partner credit and recognition in public forums (e.g., in meetings with key stakeholders and with the media).

- Be flexible and open to change as the partnership develops.

- Formalize a review of the partnership by creating an evaluation form that measures satisfaction with the partnership. This review could be done at least annually.

- Discuss and use the results of the partnership evaluation to improve the partnership.

- Discuss each partner's goals for the partnership over the long term, and what criteria will be used for continuing the partnership.

- Keep track of partnership activities, and evaluate progress and accomplishments.

- Communicate results of partnership activities with partners to show areas of success and areas for improvement.

Ending a Partnership

When a program outgrows the need for a particular partnership, or the needs change and the existing partnership is no longer crucial, meet with the partner and talk about the situation. Make sure that the parting is amicable and mutually agreed on. This leaves the window open for future opportunities to work with that organization. The partner may have other ideas on how you can continue to collaborate. If the partner expresses the desire to continue, the parties should work together to determine ways to maintain a relationship. This may or may not be the same type of partnership. It may be at a less formal or intensive level, but as long as it is mutually beneficial, it should be considered.

Engaging, Building, Expanding: An NBCCEDP Partnership Development Toolkit
Partnership Development Resources: Partnership Development Guide

March 2011

5

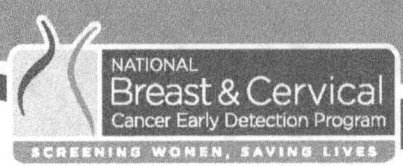

Introduction to Public and Media Relations

What Is Public Relations?

Public relations (PR) involves managing the communication between your program and your key audiences, including both the public and other stakeholders. The goals of public relations are to inform, persuade, and connect people, while building and maintaining a strong identity for your program and establishing trust among your audiences. Increased trust is the mark of effective public relations, as it can position your organization as a go-to resource for breast and cervical cancer information, education, and services, helping to foster relationships with those you are trying to reach.

Common public relations activities include media relations, social media engagement, community events, and stakeholder communications. Whether or not you choose to conduct media relations as part of your overall communications strategy, it is still vital to utilize other PR tactics to engage key audiences and get your message out.

This overview will help you determine who you are trying to reach, what you want to say, which activities best suit your goals, and how to implement some common tactics. The document covers the following:

- Audience Identification
- Message Development
- Tactics:
  - Media Relations
  - Social Media Engagement
  - Events
  - Stakeholder Communications

Audience Identification

The first step is to identify your target audience. You can define one or multiple audiences, but it is necessary to think about who the messages need to reach. This will determine the messaging and outreach strategy. Ask these questions:

- Do I want to target local or broader audiences?
- Do I want to reach the public and/or influencers (potential partners)?
- Who does this issue affect?
- Where can I find/reach my audience?
- How does my audience gather information?

By understanding your audience, you will be better equipped to shape messages that resonate with them.

Message Development

What do you want to say to your target audience? As messages are developed, focus on the most important points to serve as a foundation for the entire strategy so you don't overwhelm the audience. These points should be informative and newsworthy to attract your audience's attention. The *Talking Points* in this toolkit can help get you started. Ask these questions:

- Do I want to focus on the program as a whole, or on specific activities and goals?
- Is the goal to raise awareness or to change behavior?
- What action do I want people to take when they hear my message?
- What benefit can I offer in exchange for the action I want them to do? What reward will they get for doing what I am asking?

Introduction to Public and Media Relations

A good message should communicate clearly to your audience, be specific about what you are asking, provide motivation the audience cares about, use vivid analogies as appropriate, and be expressed at the right time by the right person. For example, when talking about your program's challenges, mention details such as who should be concerned, potential solutions to the problem, and who can affect change. Compelling messaging is critical for all communication efforts and needs to be consistent across all tactics.

Following are a few examples of ineffective vs. effective messages:

- "Our program needs partner support," is less effective than saying, "Your contribution of funds or in-kind support can help save the lives of women in your community by providing them with access to breast and cervical cancer education and screening."

- "You should partner with us," is less effective than saying, "Working with our program ensures that your contribution will directly support women in our community—including your employees and customers—and enhance your organization's presence in the community, raise your visibility as a caring corporate citizen, and heighten employee morale.

Tactics

Public relations initiatives help foster stakeholder and partner engagement by regularly informing about your program's latest activities and their impact.

1. Media Relations

A key element of PR that can amplify your efforts is media relations, with media serving as powerful allies audience and ultimately influencing behavior change.

The current media landscape is vast and includes traditional media channels such as television, newspapers, magazines and radio, as well as new media conduits like blogs and social networks. The following information can guide you in preparing for and conducting strategic media outreach that best utilizes the media channels that will effectively distribute your message.

Preparing for Media Outreach
Developing a well-honed media strategy is essential to conducting successful outreach, as it helps determine who to reach, what they should know, and how to best reach them. Once the key audience and message have been determined, the next steps are to build a media list and develop media materials. To prepare for outreach, you will also want to identify and train appropriate spokespeople.

Building a Media List
Effective media relations relies on building and maintaining strong relationships with members of the media. A media list should focus on quality rather than quantity.

- **First and foremost, DO YOUR HOMEWORK.** Reporters are far more receptive to pitches and story ideas that concentrate on topics they are either interested in or have a history of covering. Researching reporters that have written about similar topics and issues is crucial to building a mutually productive relationship.

- **Target appropriate media outlets (e.g., newspapers, broadcast news stations, and bloggers).** Because you are pitching about cancer awareness and programs, it's best to reach out to reporters who focus on health, or general reporters who cover community activities. Identify any outlets that may be sympathetic to community issues or that reach the specific audiences your program is targeting.

- **Stay organized.** It is important to stay organized so that you don't unnecessarily contact a reporter multiple times. Creating a database of contacts (i.e., in a simple spreadsheet) is the easiest way to keep track of contact information as well as pitching status.

Engaging, Building, Expanding: An NBCCEDP Partnership Development Toolkit
Partnership Development Resources: Introduction to Public and Media Relations

March 2011

2

Introduction to Public and Media Relations

Materials Development

Reporters will expect to receive a media kit to gain a deeper understanding of your issue, organization, and mission. A typical media kit can include the latest press release, a media alert, a fact sheet, biographies of key personnel/spokespersons, contact information, and talking points. These documents should be in electronic format so they can be easily emailed.

Press Release—A press release is the core foundation of a media outreach campaign because it informs the media and other stakeholders about the newsworthy issue or initiative you want to promote. Ideally, a press release should be no longer than one page and should cover only the most important points. Reporters are busy and often don't read past the first paragraph, so it is vital to include the most critical details at the top. The first sentence should answer the five "Ws"- who, what, where, when, and why. The headline should be eye-grabbing and newsworthy, with the subtitle filling in some details. For example:

....

Public/Private Partnership Brings Free Mammogram Screenings to Baltimore

October is National Breast Cancer Awareness Month

....

Please see the Appendix for guidance on how press releases are typically formatted, writing guidelines, and a sample press release.

Media Alert—A media alert (also called a media advisory) is used when there is an immediate event you would like to announce to the press. It outlines the most compelling points to draw media to cover that event. An alert should be short and the information should be bulleted, covering the five W's. Please see the appendix for a sample media alert.

Fact Sheet, Biographies, Talking Points—These standard press kit documents provide background information and facts to help reporters ensure accuracy in their coverage. To be used as supporting documents for all activities, they can remain largely unchanged because they outline constant facts rather than news or updates. Like the media alert, these documents should be bulleted.

Training Spokespeople

If you are offering spokespeople as part of your media outreach, it is important to train them on key messages and the goals. As part of your training, consider practicing media interviewing skills and techniques, such as delivering messages in a question-and-answer format, in mock exercises that are recorded and replayed for instant analysis and feedback.

Keep in mind, though, that a spokesperson is anyone who speaks on your behalf, whether while staffing a booth at an event, at a conference, or to media. They all need to know key messages and be prepared. Spokespeople should be comfortable with your messages, program, and any sensitive topics before participating in program outreach.

Conducting Media Outreach

Once the materials are assembled, spokespersons are trained, and the media list is set (if appropriate), you are ready to conduct media outreach. Your outreach efforts will vary depending on the type of placement you want. For example, you will have to write the content for op-eds, which are written opinions of a named writer who is usually unaffiliated with the newspaper's editorial board. Similarly, you will also write the content for letters to the editor, which usually have specific parameters that can be found on the outlet's website or by calling them directly. For an editorial, you will usually have to meet with the outlet's editorial board to discuss your story idea. For a general article, you can just contact the reporter or editor directly to "pitch" your story idea.

For a press release or media alert, there are multiple distribution options. You can develop a media list through Internet research or a media service such as Vocus (www.vocuspr.com) or Cision (http://us.cision.com) and distribute the information yourself, or engage a press release distribution service such as PR Newswire (www.prnewswire.com) or Marketwire (www.marketwire.com).

Engaging, Building, Expanding: An NBCCEDP Partnership Development Toolkit
Partnership Development Resources: Introduction to Public and Media Relations

March 2011

3

Introduction to Public and Media Relations

Important tips to remember when pitching:

- **Email is best.** Most reporters prefer to receive pitches through email, but it can be helpful to follow up with a phone call.

- **Make it newsworthy.** Pitching a story is competitive; members of the media can get hundreds of pitches a day. Because of this, make sure your story is newsworthy (relevant and of widespread interest) to give you an advantage over the competition. When pitching, timing is important. Try to relate the pitch to recent news events, adding to its newsworthiness.

- **Keep it short.** Keep the messages brief. Don't give too much information away in the pitch as it should stimulate a reporter's appetite for more information.

- **Tailor pitches.** Reporters and editors appreciate a more personal pitch, which demonstrates that you are familiar with their interests and previous work.

- **Offer an interview.** Offer an interview with a spokesperson or key expert.

- **Become a resource.** Should a reporter, editor, or producer choose not to use your story idea, offer yourself as a resource for future stories. This can help in maintaining a mutually beneficial relationship.

- **Keep track.** Stay on top of coverage through media monitoring. Google Alerts can be a useful tool in managing placements; Google will search and email news stories as they happen based on your search terms. You can set up alerts at www.google.com/alerts. Try keywords such as:

  - Your organization's name
  - Your organization's acronym (if applicable)
  - The names and acronyms of your partners
  - "Breast cancer"
  - "Cervical cancer"

2. Social Media Engagement

Though you may be using traditional media (e.g., print, TV, or radio) to reach your audience, it is worth exploring some level of social media engagement (e.g., blogs, Twitter, or Facebook) as part of an overall media outreach strategy. Social media reflects a fundamental shift in the way we behave and communicate, creating new opportunities for outreach and message placement. With 58% of online users having established a social network profile, social media is becoming more widespread and mainstream.

You don't need a lot of experience in this area to have an impact; it can be as easy as establishing a Facebook page, creating a Twitter handle, or uploading photos to Flickr. These networks can be a fast, easy, and free way to disseminate timely information to many people— 400 million people are on Facebook and 75 million people visit Twitter each month. If your organization currently blocks access to social media websites, you may need to request special access to start a social media program.

- **Facebook.** (www.facebook.com) Perhaps the most comprehensive social medium, Facebook is an effective platform to help build a community. It serves as an online meeting place where you and your followers can share photos, videos, events, and post messages.

- **Twitter.** (www.twitter.com/signup) A great way to initiate a conversation by sharing information in real time with millions of users. For example, you can "tweet" live from an event, which will help generate excitement and interest.

- **Flickr.** (www.flickr.com) A photo sharing site that can help round out your social media engagement by adding a visual element to your campaign. You can post photos from your events, or ask women in your community to share their photos (e.g., from a local Komen walk).

Facebook, Twitter, and Flickr are just a few of the many social media websites. Find the sites that are most relevant to your program and audiences.

Another social media tactic is to connect with relevant bloggers, who you can find through sites like www.alltop.com and www.blogsearch.google.com. Like print reporters, bloggers respond mainly to story ideas that reflect their interests, so you need to do your research.

Engaging, Building, Expanding: An NBCCEDP Partnership Development Toolkit
Partnership Development Resources: Introduction to Public and Media Relations

March 2011

4

Introduction to Public and Media Relations

As you engage in social media tactics, it is important to understand that you cannot always control the conversation among constituents. You might consider developing internal guidelines for engagement and monitoring of social media activities to be prepared for both positive and negative feedback.

3. Events

Events are an effective way to quickly draw attention and bring your message to life. Whether you host a rally with speakers, an intimate luncheon with influencers, or organize a walk-a-thon, an event itself can generate publicity and can connect you directly with your audience. To best reach your targeted audience, ask:

- Where does my audience go?
- What do they like to do?
- Is the goal of the event to attract the media or influencers?
- Is this newsworthy?
- How big should the event be?
- Is this timed appropriately?
- What speakers should participate?
- What kinds of logistics are involved?

4. Stakeholder Communications

Engaging stakeholders and influencers through internal communications is vital to maintaining their support. These communication efforts can be more specific and tailored to your audience. For example, newsletters can be less formal, and can tell more personal stories about your organization, successes, and latest activities. In addition, keep a database of stakeholders and contact them about once a month to provide updates on your program, and see what they are working on. These calls can help nurture lasting and more personal relationships.

SAMPLE NEWSLETTER BLURB

Below is a sample newsletter blurb about partnerships that can be used to remind stakeholders about your program's needs and the benefits of partnering.

Partner with Us
As you know, **[Program Name]**, in partnership with the National Breast and Cervical Cancer Early Detection Program, provides breast and cervical cancer education as well as free and low-cost services to low-income, uninsured, and underserved women. With more women in need of services than in years past, we need greater resources now, more than ever before. Partners—including local businesses, corporations, health care providers, faith-based organizations, community-based organizations, and many others—can provide a range of in-kind and monetary contributions to help women in our community access critically needed breast and cervical cancer-related services. Our program has a range of unique needs and can benefit from partnerships of any size or scale—no contribution is too small. If you are interested in learning more about how you can work with us to improve the health of women, please contact us at **[email/phone]**.

Engaging, Building, Expanding: An NBCCEDP Partnership Development Toolkit
Partnership Development Resources: Introduction to Public and Media Relations

March 2011

5

Introduction to Public and Media Relations

Appendix

Typical Press Release Format:

- Place the phrase "For Immediate Release" and the date on the upper left margin.

- Below this phrase or on the right margin, place your contact person's name, phone number, and email.

- Compose a short headline that clearly describes the news release content and grabs the reader's attention. Center it in bold type on the page. Place concise secondary subheads in italics below the main headline.

- Begin the first paragraph with your dateline. The dateline identifies where the news originated. For example, "MADISON, WI—The Madison Health Department launched a new program today to increase access to treatment for breast and cervical cancer through a special Medicaid option program."

- First paragraph: Provide the date, time, and other time-critical information related to your activities. Concisely summarize the facts—who, what, when, where, and why—in the first paragraph.

- Second paragraph: Insert a quote from a leader within your organization, such as the director or a project head, about the event or program. Be sure to identify the source of all quotes. Make sure that the quote content explains and enhances the story, and that there is a clear relationship between the person quoted and the story. Try to limit the number of quotes to no more than two people.

- Third paragraph: Include details on the event and the program.

- Final paragraph: Covers basic organizational information, such as who you are and the history of the event or program. If you have a list of member organizations, sponsors, or other partners, list them in an attachment rather than incorporating that information into the text of the release. This makes it easier for a reporter or editor to review.

- If your release goes beyond one page, type "-more-" at the bottom of the first page. Keep the release to a maximum of two pages, but strive for one.

- At the end of your release, type "###" or "-30-" to indicate the end of the copy.

Press Release Writing Guidelines:

- Use short, declarative sentences and double-space the lines. Make sure to use an active verb and the word "today" in your first sentence.

- Avoid the use of jargon and explain any acronyms at their first use, e.g., "The Centers for Disease Control and Prevention (CDC)..." Avoid "puff" words and phrases such as "exciting," "very large," "monumental." Be as clear and concrete as possible in your descriptions.

- Link the facts of the project or event to an important issue or need in your local community. Using real-life examples helps make the human connection. Highlight benefits of your work to the community.

- Review the release for clarity and flow, and be sure that all words and names are spelled correctly.

Be sure to include a quote from the program's leader, as reporters will often use quotes they find in a release. At the end of the release, add a boiler plate—a short paragraph about the organization. Here is an example from NBCCEDP:

....

The National Breast and Cervical Cancer Early Detection Program of the Centers for Disease Control and Prevention provides public education, free and low-cost breast and cervical cancer screenings, and diagnostic services to low-income, uninsured, and underserved women.

....

Engaging, Building, Expanding: An NBCCEDP Partnership Development Toolkit
Partnership Development Resources: Introduction to Public and Media Relations

March 2011   6

Introduction to Public and Media Relations

NBCCEDP Press Release Sample—Partner Collaboration on Local Screening Event
NOTE: This sample is based on a fictitious scenario and does not depict real people, organizations, or activities.

SAMPLE PRESS RELEASE

FOR IMMEDIATE RELEASE
October 1, 2009
Contact: Jane Smith, jsmith@domain.com, 555-123-4567

Public/Private Partnership Brings Free Mammogram Screenings to Baltimore
October is National Breast Cancer Awareness Month

Baltimore, MD—Throughout National Breast Cancer Awareness Month in October, the WomenCare Breast and Cervical Cancer Screening Program and Paulson Grocery Stores are partnering to offer free breast cancer screenings to low-income (at or below 250% of the federal poverty level), uninsured, and undeserved women 40 to 64 years old in Baltimore City and County.

"Getting a mammogram that could save your life takes about as long as a trip to the grocery store," said WomenCare's Program Director Susie Cue. "Paulson's generous contribution of time and money are making these events possible."

This is the first year WomenCare and Paulson are working together to raise awareness of the importance of getting mammograms in the fight to reduce the breast cancer death rate. Baltimore County has the highest breast cancer death rate in the state, and Maryland is ranked seventh in the country. "At Paulson, our commitment to the community is a cornerstone of our business," said John Peters, Mid-Atlantic Regional Manager of Operations for Paulson Grocery Stores. "We are thrilled to be able to help our neighborhoods address the critical need for mammograms."

Program-eligible women (as defined above) will need to bring valid photo identification with them, and can expect that their appointment will take about 30 minutes. For women who are not able to have a mammogram onsite, WomenCare will have staff available to help schedule future appointments with medical providers at a mutually convenient time and place.

"Getting screened at one of WomenCare's events last year saved my life," said Sandra Dee, a Baltimore resident of more than 40 years. "I would never have known I had cancer if I didn't go, since I had been without insurance for some time."

On the following days and times, free mammograms will be available onsite for qualifying women at the following Paulson locations:

	Saturday 10/9/09	Sunday 10/10/09	Saturday 10/23/09	Sunday 10/24/09
8 a.m. – 12 p.m.	Towson, MD	Woodberry, MD	Woodlawn, MD	Rosedale, MD
1 p.m. – 5 p.m.	Parkville, MD	Baltimore City, MD	Owings Mills, MD	White Marsh, MD

— more —

Engaging, Building, Expanding: An NBCCEDP Partnership Development Toolkit
Partnership Development Resources: Introduction to Public and Media Relations

March 2011

7

SAMPLE PRESS RELEASE (continued)

Since WomenCare's inception in 1992, the program has screened more than 20,000 women, and has diagnosed more than 300 women through breast or cervical cancer screening using federal, state, and partner support.

The WomenCare Breast and Cervical Cancer Screening Program, a program of the National Breast and Cervical Cancer Early Detection Program, provides public education, free and low-cost breast and cervical cancer screenings, and diagnostic services to low-income, uninsured, and underserved women. Visit www.WomenCare.state.us for more information.

Paulson Grocery Stores, established in 1910, is one of the leading grocery chains in the United States. The Company operates 5,462 stores in 30 states and the District of Columbia. A commitment to local communities and businesses is a part of Paulson's mission. Most Paulson locations have full-service pharmacies and all stores feature fresh and local products.

###

Engaging, Building, Expanding: An NBCCEDP Partnership Development Toolkit
Partnership Development Resources: Introduction to Public and Media Relations

March 2011

8

Introduction to Public and Media Relations

NBCCEDP Media Alert Sample—Partner Collaboration on Local Screening Event
NOTE: This sample is based on a fictitious scenario and does not depict real people, organizations, or activities.

SAMPLE MEDIA ALERT

For Immediate Release: October 1, 2009
Contact: Jane Smith, jsmith@domain.com, 555-123-4567

WHO: The WomenCare Breast and Cervical Cancer Screening Program and Paulson Grocery Stores

WHAT: Free mammogram screenings throughout the month of October to low-income (at or below 250% of the federal poverty level), uninsured, and underserved women 40 to 64 years old in Baltimore City and County.

WHEN and WHERE: Below are the dates and times at participating Paulson stores:

	Saturday 10/9/09	Sunday 10/10/09	Saturday 10/23/09	Sunday 10/24/09
8 a.m. – 12 p.m.	Towson, MD	Woodberry, MD	Woodlawn, MD	Rosedale, MD
1 p.m. – 5 p.m.	Parkville, MD	Baltimore City, MD	Owings Mills, MD	White Marsh, MD

The WomenCare Breast and Cervical Cancer Screening Program, a program of the National Breast and Cervical Cancer Early Detection Program, provides public education, free and low-cost breast and cervical cancer screenings, and diagnostic services to low-income, uninsured, and underserved women. Visit www.womenmatter.state.us for more information.

Paulson Grocery Stores, established in 1910, is one of the leading grocery chains in the United States. The Company operates 5,462 stores in 30 states and the District of Columbia. A commitment to local communities and businesses is a part of Paulson's mission. Most Paulson locations have full-service pharmacies and all stores feature fresh and local products.

###

Engaging, Building, Expanding: An NBCCEDP Partnership Development Toolkit
Partnership Development Resources: Introduction to Public and Media Relations

March 2011

9

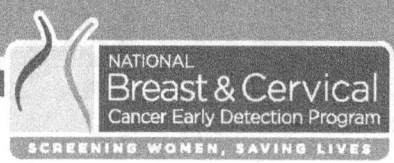

Talking Points

The talking points below provide simple language that programs can use to communicate with potential partners about the National Breast and Cervical Cancer Early Detection Program (NBCCEDP), and about the importance and benefits of partnerships. Use only the messages you need and tailor them to your particular audience, depending on what you are trying to accomplish. Add emotional appeal by including specific information about the women in your community or state, the consequences of missed screenings, and your program's impact on saving women's lives. Suggestions on ways to customize the messages are included below.

Core Message

With the support of program partners, the National Breast and Cervical Cancer Early Detection Program can continue providing critically needed breast and cervical cancer education, screening, and diagnostic services to low-income, uninsured, and underserved women in the United States, for free or at a minimal cost.

SUPPORTING MESSAGE 1

In 1990, Congress established NBCCEDP to aid in the fight against breast and cervical cancers, which claim the lives of thousands of women each year.

- Breast and cervical cancer screenings and early detection save lives.
- NBCCEDP was established to serve low-income, uninsured, and underserved women in the U.S. who lack access to vital medical and education services.
- Breast cancer is most treatable when detected early through regular screenings.
- Cervical cancer is highly preventable with regular screenings, and treatable when found early.
- Regular breast and cervical cancer screenings protect women in the prime of their lives, allowing them to maintain productivity and continue as primary caregivers for their families.

CUSTOMIZE YOUR MESSAGE

Develop a message about the history of your program (e.g., when your program was established, and unique populations served).

SUPPORTING MESSAGE 2

NBCCEDP provides consumer education, free and low-cost breast and cervical cancer screenings, and diagnostic services to women in need.

- For the past 20 years, NBCCEDP has served more than 3.7 million women and provided more than 9.2 million screening examinations.[1]
- An estimated 8%–11% of U.S. women of screening age are eligible to receive NBCCEDP services.
- NBCCEDP funds programs in all 50 states, the District of Columbia, five U.S. territories, and 12 American Indian/Alaska Native tribal organizations.

CUSTOMIZE YOUR MESSAGE

Develop a message about how many women your program served either from its inception or in the past year.

1

Talking Points

Federal funding alone cannot fully sustain NBCCEDP programs—support from partners is needed.

- Programs are required to match every $3 of federal funds they receive with $1 of non-federal resources (monetary or in-kind). Further, matching funds annually must equal or exceed the amount the program was contributing prior to its initial award of federal funds.
- If the amount of federal funding remains constant, the amount of funding received by programs each year for screening and education does not go as far due to inflation.
- Some states, which often provide significant funding to programs, are cutting or significantly reducing their support due to financial crises.
- More women are in need of NBCCEDP's services than in years past. Programs need resources now, more than ever before.

> CUSTOMIZE YOUR MESSAGE
>
> Consider quantifying the decrease in state/partner funding, or the amount of funding that your program needs, if this information is available (e.g., X number of women cannot be screened or served because of the decrease in funding).

As a partner with NBCCEDP's programs, you can provide a range of in-kind and monetary contributions and support to help women access critically needed breast and cervical cancer-related services.

- Programs are currently seeking support from diverse partners, including partners like you: local businesses, corporations, health care providers, community-based organizations, faith-based organizations, and many others.
- No contribution is too small.
- In addition to direct funding, your help is needed with in-kind contributions, such as consumer education, provider education, printing, translation services, recruitment, fundraising, meeting facility provision, advocacy, and other activities and services.
- Your organization can support NBCCEDP programs by encouraging volunteerism among your employees or adopting policies that promote and support screening.

> CUSTOMIZE YOUR MESSAGE
>
> Think about what your program can specifically benefit from and tailor these messages accordingly. In addition, if you know how many women can be served with $1,000 or some other monetary amount, insert that information here.

Engaging, Building, Expanding: An NBCCEDP Partnership Development Toolkit
Partnership Development Resources: Talking Points

March 2011

2

Talking Points

SUPPORTING MESSAGE 5

Partnering with NBCCEDP programs provides many benefits.

- Providing resources to NBCCEDP programs ensures that your contribution will directly benefit women in your community—including your employees or customers.

- Partnering with NBCCEDP programs gives your organization a presence in the community, raises your organization's visibility as a caring corporate citizen, and improves employee morale.

- Partnering with NBCCEDP programs links your organization to a credible and highly respected government breast and cervical cancer program.

- Partnering with NBCCEDP programs can lead to numerous marketing, public relations, and networking opportunities.

CUSTOMIZE YOUR MESSAGE

Breast and cervical cancers affect everyone. Specify which groups they affect as relevant to the partner, such as their members, customers, employees, and/or other constituents.

Add specific state benefits that may apply, such as tax benefits.

Look at *Ways to Work With Partners* in this toolkit for additional suggestions on customizing appeals for specific types of organizations.

References

1 Centers for Disease Control and Prevention, National Breast and Cervical Cancer Early Detection Program. *Minimum Data Elements.* April 2010.

Engaging, Building, Expanding: An NBCCEDP Partnership Development Toolkit
Partnership Development Resources: Talking Points

March 2011

3

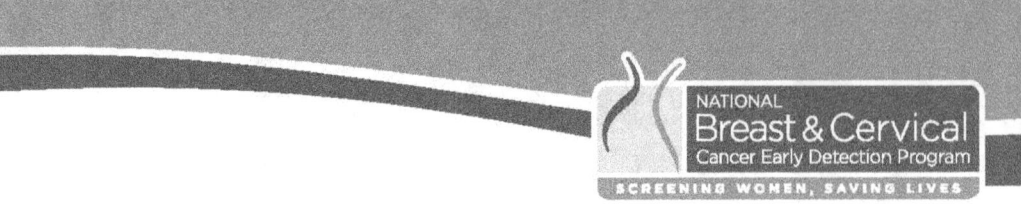

Making Your Case

When communicating with potential and existing partners, you may need to express the needs and impact of your program, as well as the value of partner support, in different ways depending on the type of organization. Below are suggestions for effectively educating partners about your program and the great work you are doing, and for persuading partners to provide funding or other resources.

Prepare

- **Do advance research.** Spend some time looking into the partner organization and person you will be speaking with, how they define value, and the best way to communicate (e.g., formal presentation, phone conversation, email).

- **Develop your key messages.** Create a list of potential questions and prepare your answers (review the questions and answers in *Sample Answers to Common Partner Questions* in this toolkit). Make sure your answers are short, to the point, and most importantly, convey the intended message. Try to avoid technical language and buzz words. Practice your key messages, but don't try to memorize them word for word—relying on memory can cause you to freeze up. Review the *Talking Points* and *Sample Elevator Speech* in this toolkit for more information.

- **Be mindful of timing.** There are certain times of year when information about breast and cervical cancer will be top of mind due to national awareness months (e.g., National Breast Cancer Awareness Month in October and Cervical Cancer Awareness Month in January). These months are perfect opportunities to talk to potential partners. You can emphasize that their timely support may lead to a favorable news story or publicity highlighting their association with your program.

- **Consider the messenger.** Does someone at your organization have an existing relationship with a partner? If so, consider tapping their input and influence. Gaining their feedback on outreach approaches and messages are great ways to help ensure that the right messages are being conveyed. You can also consider engaging them to carry your message forward to the partner. In doing so, make sure they are prepared with your key messages and familiar with your program's materials.

Engage

- **Help partners understand your previous successes and the importance of your services to the community.** Potential partners will want to know they are supporting an accomplished program, so be sure to articulate clearly what your program has achieved in the past. Emphasize the importance of educating women in the community about breast and cervical cancer; share information on the need for breast and cervical cancer screening and diagnostics; or provide statistics on the number of women in your community who qualify for National Breast and Cervical Cancer Early Detection Program (NBCCEDP) services and the number of women who depend on your program's services.

- **Don't forget to share the bad stories too.** It is, of course, important to highlight your program's successes; however, it is equally important to share information about the challenges your program faces. Consider providing information on the number of women placed on waiting lists, the number women who qualify but are not active with the program, decreases in services offered, and other challenges.

- **Be specific.** When communicating with partners, ask for something specific and provide a specific statement of what you will deliver. This may facilitate and streamline the process. Review *Ways to Work With Partners* in this toolkit to help generate ideas.

Making Your Case

- **Highlight the community focus.** Explain that the resources they provide are used to help women in your community. This is a unique selling point, as some partners may feel strongly about having their support go directly back to the community.

- **Emphasize other community partners.** With their permission, build awareness of the other partners who are pitching in and working together to sustain an important community program. This may create a bandwagon effect and help persuade your potential partner to support the program.

- **Be creative in how you present data.** Share the data your program routinely collects, as it likely is new and powerful to partners and establishes credibility. Also consider presenting the data in different ways—can you calculate how many cases of cervical cancers were prevented; how many lives saved; or how many years of life women gained? Such data can also be used by partners to help with advocacy efforts.

- **Illustrate your program's importance to the community.** Your program provides key services to your community. Paint a picture for potential partners of what would be missing if your program could not provide breast and cervical cancer services.

Recognize

- **Publicly recognize partners where appropriate.** Develop a plan to recognize each partner's contributions to the success of your program. Check with partners before publicly recognizing them to ensure they are comfortable with your plan.

- **Follow up with partner organizations to share results from their contributions.** Partners may feel buoyed learning the impact of their support to your organization. Did their monetary donation allow for additional mammograms? Did the donated advertisement space in the newspaper bring more people to an event? Did a new group of women seek out the program services because of a partner's outreach efforts? If so, share this with the partners to reinforce how meaningful their support is to your program and to demonstrate accountability. Refer to the *Thank You Letter* and *Recognition Certificate* in this toolkit for ideas.

Engaging, Building, Expanding: An NBCCEDP Partnership Development Toolkit
Partnership Development Resources: Making Your Case

March 2011

2

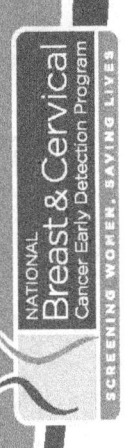

SCREENING WOMEN. SAVING LIVES

NATIONAL
Breast & Cervical
Cancer Early Detection Program

Ways to Work With Partners

TYPE OF PARTNER	POTENTIAL ASSETS	WAYS PARTNERS CAN HELP
Corporate		
• Insurance companies • Large local employers • Local franchises of national companies (e.g., department stores, food chains, or pharmacy/drug stores) • Local retail businesses • Local professional services companies • Restaurants and bars • Salons • Sports teams	• Access to external and internal communication channels • Customer and employee base • Fundraising and events expertise • In-kind contributions • Marketing and outreach resources • Monetary contributions • Promotional tie-ins	• Promote NBCCEDP services (online, in-store, through mailers, etc.), especially during cancer awareness observance months • Conduct public education or screening initiatives among customers and employees • Host fundraiser/themed events with percentage of sales going to program • Collaborate on in-kind partnerships (e.g., partnership to provide event space or medical supplies; prizes or refreshments for meetings or trainings) • Provide pro-bono professional services (printing, advertising, communications support, etc.) • Provide monetary support through community relations projects, corporate grants, or philanthropy programs to meet matching fund requirements
Local Government Entities		
• Cancer registries • CDC's Comprehensive Cancer Control Program • Elected officials • Federal agencies' offices of women's health (e.g., HHS, FDA, or NIH) • Indian Health Services • Medicare • NCI's Cancer Information Service • Public transportation • State and local offices for aging or minority health • State and local public health agencies/initiatives (e.g., chronic disease, family planning, emergency response, infectious disease)	• Access to external and internal communication channels • Audience expertise • Data and statistics • Established programming and infrastructure • Facilities for meetings and/or screenings • In-kind contributions • Public education materials • Subject matter/audience expertise • Volunteers	• Cross-promote programs through websites, newsletters, and email blasts • Conduct targeted outreach to priority target audiences • Advise on cultural sensitivities • Provide assistance with research and evaluation • Coordinate outreach efforts to include breast and cervical cancer information • Conduct inreach to refer priority populations into the NBCCEDP program • Provide a community health worker (or funding for one) to do targeted outreach • Offer facilities (rooms or offices) for meetings, trainings, or patient screening/consultation • Participate in advisory committees or coalitions to support breast and cervical cancer screening and education

Engaging, Building, Expanding: An NBCCEDP Partnership Development Toolkit
Partnership Development Resources: Ways to Work With Partners

March 2011

1

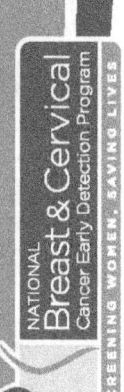

Ways to Work With Partners

TYPE OF PARTNER	POTENTIAL ASSETS	WAYS PARTNERS CAN HELP
Community-based Organizations		
• Cultural groups (e.g., cultural societies, sororities) • Civic organizations (e.g., Lion's Club, YWCA, United Way) • Health organizations focused on priority audiences	• Audience expertise • Credibility and reputation • Established programming and infrastructure • Facilities for meetings and/ or screenings • Funding mechanisms for channeling monetary donations from the public • Fundraising and events expertise • In-kind donations • Language proficiency/translation resources • Mailing lists • Marketing and outreach resources • Member base • Monetary contributions • Spokespeople • Statistics and data • Volunteers	• Conduct targeted outreach to priority audiences • Advise on cultural sensitivities • Refer patients to treatment, survivorship, and other cancer-related services • Cross-promote programs through websites, newsletters, and email blasts • Offer facilities (rooms or offices) for meetings, trainings, or patient screening/consultation • Form an indirect partnership with an organization that has a mechanism for taking monetary donations from benefactors and applying them to breast and cervical cancer-related services for women in need • Host a fundraiser with NBCCEDP that supports both organizations • Provide individualized support for patients (e.g., transportation, translation) • Translate existing materials to enable recruitment of high priority/ hard-to-reach audiences • Coordinate with NBCCEDP's efforts during cancer awareness months • Solicit donation of services from members and their contacts • Provide grant funding for screening women to meet matching fund requirements • Collaborate with advocacy groups and other partners to attest to/quantify level of need • Provide assistance with research and evaluation • Provide a community health worker (or funding for one) to do targeted outreach • Participate in advisory committees or coalitions to support breast and cervical cancer screening and education

Engaging, Building, Expanding: An NBCCEDP Partnership Development Toolkit
Partnership Development Resources: Ways to Work With Partners

March 2011

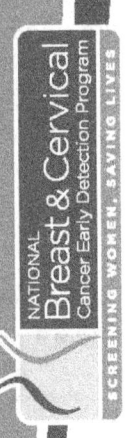

NATIONAL
Breast & Cervical
Cancer Early Detection Program
SCREENING WOMEN. SAVING LIVES.

Ways to Work With Partners

TYPE OF PARTNER	POTENTIAL ASSETS	WAYS PARTNERS CAN HELP
Faith-based Organizations		
• Nonprofit organizations with religious affiliations (e.g., Salvation Army, Catholic Charities) • Places of worship such as churches, synagogues, or mosques	• Credibility and reputation • Facilities for meetings and/or screenings • Marketing and outreach resources • Member base	• Conduct public education or screening initiatives among congregants • Conduct targeted outreach to priority audiences that are among their membership • Offer facilities (rooms or offices) for meetings, trainings, or patient screening/consultation • Solicit donation of services from members and their contacts • Host a fundraiser with NBCCEDP that supports both organizations • Coordinate with NBCCEDP's efforts during cancer awareness months • Participate in advisory committees or coalitions to support breast and cervical cancer screening and education
NBCCEDP's National Partners		
• American Cancer Society • Avon Foundation for Women • Susan G. Komen for the Cure®	• Credibility and reputation • Established programming and infrastructure • Fundraising and events expertise • Marketing and outreach resources • Monetary contributions • Professional development (workshops, etc) • Resources for advocating on NBCCEDP's behalf • Statistics and data	• Cross-promote programs through websites, newsletters, and email blasts • Collaborate on fundraising initiatives • Conduct targeted outreach to priority populations • Refer patients to treatment, survivorship, and other cancer-related services • Coordinate with program's efforts during cancer awareness months • Provide grant funding for screening women or in-kind donations to meet matching fund requirements • Team up on grant applications • Provide training resources for professional development (e.g., data management, grant writing, marketing, and outreach) • Participate in advisory committees or coalitions to support breast and cervical cancer screening and education • Advocate for NBCCEDP on the state and national levels • Provide assistance with research and evaluation

3

Engaging, Building, Expanding: An NBCCEDP Partnership Development Toolkit
Partnership Development Resources: Ways to Work With Partners

March 2011

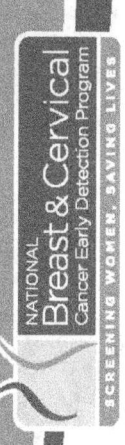

Ways to Work With Partners

TYPE OF PARTNER	POTENTIAL ASSETS	WAYS PARTNERS CAN HELP
Cancer Groups		
• National nonprofits (e.g., National Breast Cancer Foundation or National Coalition for Cervical Cancer) • Local nonprofits (e.g., chapters of national organizations or grassroots organizations with local focus)	• Credibility and reputation • Facilities for meetings and/ or screenings • Fundraising and events expertise • Funding mechanisms for channeling monetary donations from the public • Marketing and outreach resources • Member base • Monetary contributions • Spokespeople • Statistics and data	• Offer facilities (rooms or offices) for meetings, trainings, or patient screening/consultation • Collaborate on fundraising initiatives • Form an indirect partnership with an organization that has a mechanism for taking monetary donations from benefactors and applying them to breast and cervical cancer-related services for women in need • Cross-promote programs through websites, newsletters, and email blasts • Coordinate with program's efforts during cancer awareness months • Collaborate on outreach and public education activities, such as creating a traveling exhibit that communicates the common messages among partners • Collaborate on a media event to raise awareness • Coordinate on individual initiatives to maximize efficiency and avoid duplication of effort • Collaborate with advocacy groups and other partners to attest to/quantify level of need • Participate in advisory committees or coalitions to support breast and cervical cancer screening and education
Cancer Alliances and Coalitions		
	• Access to respective participants' organizations • Credibility and reputation • Professional networks • Spokespeople • Statistics and data	• Offer access to participants' respective organizations' resources (in-kind or monetary) • Advise on medical, advocacy, and social topics related to breast and cervical cancer • Provide unique perspectives on local issues related to screening women for breast and cervical cancer • Collaborate to plan events and other public education initiatives • Support local advocacy efforts

Engaging, Building, Expanding: An NBCCEDP Partnership Development Toolkit
Partnership Development Resources: Ways to Work With Partners

March 2011

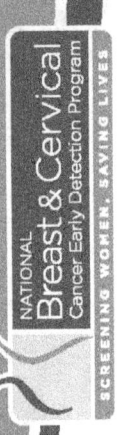

Ways to Work With Partners

TYPE OF PARTNER	POTENTIAL ASSETS	WAYS PARTNERS CAN HELP
Medical Service Providers		
• For-profit providers • Hospital systems • Managed care organizations • Nonprofit providers • Private practice providers • Professional associations whose members are health care providers	• Access to members (professional associations) • Access to patients • Equipment, supplies, and/or facilities for screening • Health care providers for screening • Knowledge of clinical topics • Software and technology • Spokespeople (patients and health professionals)	• Conduct public education or screening initiatives • Conduct inreach to refer specific populations into NBCCEDP programs • Cross-promote programs through websites, newsletters, and email blasts • Provide NBCCEDP program information to medical service providers (members) through Continuing Education curricula • Offer facilities (rooms or offices) for meetings, trainings, or patient screening/consultation • Provide pro-bono screening or counseling services, especially in hard-to-reach audiences • Refer patients to clinical trials providing an option for treatment when appropriate • Advise on medical topics related to breast and cervical cancer, including feedback on public education materials • Create a medical advisory board to offer counsel on clinical protocols and provide consultation on complicated cases • Connect NBCCEDP program with recipients of services for testimonials • Participate in advisory committees or coalitions to support breast and cervical cancer screening and education • Provide access to software and technology (e.g., those that analyze patient care from medical records)
Universities		
	• Equipment, supplies, and/or facilities for screening • Interns/volunteers • Knowledge of clinical topics • Language proficiency/translation resources • Marketing and outreach resources • Monetary contributions • Statistics and data	• Offer facilities (rooms or offices) for meetings, trainings, or patient screening/consultation • Provide assistance with research and evaluation (possibly a collaborative effort with a department of public health, journalism, or marketing) • Keep NBCCEDP informed of clinical trials that may provide treatment options for patients • Translate existing materials to enable recruitment of high priority/hard-to-reach audiences • Provide a community health worker, intern, or fellow (or funding for one) • Provide monetary contributions through grants and other funding mechanisms • Participate in advisory committees or coalitions to support breast and cervical cancer screening and education

Engaging, Building, Expanding: An NBCCEDP Partnership Development Toolkit
Partnership Development Resources: Ways to Work With Partners

March 2011

5

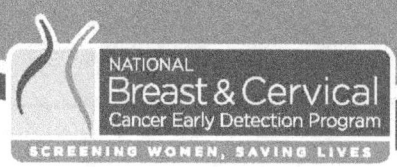

Working with Our National Partners

The National Breast and Cervical Cancer Early Detection Program (NBCCEDP) has established partnerships with a number of prominent national organizations. Below are overviews and specific partnership suggestions for the American Cancer Society, the Avon Foundation for Women, and Susan G. Komen for the Cure®—organizations that have been particularly active partners with NBCCEDP and its funded programs.

The American Cancer Society

The American Cancer Society (the Society) is a community-based, voluntary health organization dedicated to eliminating cancer as a major health problem by preventing cancer through research, education, advocacy, and service. With more than two million volunteers nationwide, the Society is one of the oldest and largest voluntary health organizations in the U.S. Through its *The Official Sponsor Of Birthdays* campaign, the Society is working to create a world with more birthdays and less cancer by helping people stay well, get well, find cures, and fight back.

As the delivery of health care continues to change, the Society is working with partners in all sectors of the health care system so that all individuals are offered a full range of preventive services. Specifically, the Society works in partnership with many public and private organizations in diverse settings to increase awareness about cancer and the importance of early detection, as well as overcoming the barriers to screening methods, such as mammograms.

The Society has also identified advocacy as one of its top corporate priorities and works nationwide to promote beneficial policies, laws, and regulations for those affected by cancer.

Specific Ways to Partner

- **Support the Society's Advocacy Efforts:** The Society's Cancer Action Network is a longstanding and valued advocacy partner for many NBCCEDP programs. To support the Society's advocacy efforts to expand local program funding, your program can equip the Society with compelling data and statistics

that supplement what NBCCEDP provides at the national level. More information about the Cancer Action Network is available online at www.acscan.org.

- **Judiciously Utilize Funds Obtained through Advocacy:** Because it requires significant effort to obtain additional funding for NBCCEDP programs, it is important that you have a plan for using the funds within the allowable time frame, if and when funding is secured.

- **Share Impact of Advocacy Successes:** NBCCEDP programs should report back to the Society on the successes accomplished through increased funding from advocacy. *Did the waiting list shrink by half? How many women's lives were saved as a result of early detection screenings from increased funding?* Anecdotal and quantitative evidence of how state funds improved the lives of women can be persuasive for the Society's future advocacy outreach efforts on your behalf.

- **Build Outreach Capacity:** The Society can provide a range of support for your outreach efforts to target populations, including women who are rarely or have never been screened. For example, the Society offers educational resources and tools to support community health workers who conduct targeted recruitment. In addition, you can leverage the Society's community partnerships to strengthen outreach to populations in need of breast and cervical cancer screenings.

- **Utilize the Society's Research-based Resources:** The Society conducts various types of research, including state-by-state mammography trend evaluation, as well as identification of evidence-based interventions to address disparities and new ways to reach rarely or never screened women. You can utilize guidance from these resources in program planning efforts.

- **Collaborate through Local Coalitions and Advisory Boards:** NBCCEDP programs can lead or participate in coalitions or advisory boards, which may include the Society, bringing together a range of people with diverse skill sets and areas of expertise.

- **Communicate on a Regular Basis:** As with other nonprofit organizations, turnover can be high at affiliate chapters. NBCCEDP programs are encouraged to regularly communicate with affiliates and reintroduce themselves as needed to keep their partnerships strong.

For more information about partnering with the Society, please call 1-800-227-2345 to be connected with a state or local contact.

The Avon Foundation for Women

The Avon Foundation for Women (the Foundation) is a corporate-affiliated foundation that focuses on improving the lives of women and their families. This mission is brought to life through two key initiatives: the *Speak Out Against Domestic Violence* program and the *Avon Breast Cancer Crusade*. To date, the Foundation has raised more than $725 million and has awarded hundreds of millions of dollars in grants to community-based organizations supporting both causes, including nonprofit breast health programs, leading cancer centers, and global organizations. Funds have been awarded for education and awareness, screening and diagnosis, access to treatment, support services, and scientific research. The Foundation's funding decisions are informed by the Avon Foundation Scientific Advisory Board, which evaluates proposed beneficiary projects and provides strategic direction for its breast cancer programs.

The Foundation supports breast health programs in the U.S. through the Avon Breast Health Outreach Program (BHOP). The Avon BHOP coordinates grants to 130 to 150 community-based breast health programs that support outreach, promote breast health education, and refer women to programs like the NBCCEDP for screening services and follow-up care in partnership with local medical providers. The Foundation *cannot fund direct costs of patient care or treatment*, including those offered through the NBCCEDP. However, a number of other recommended ways to work together are listed below. Details on funding guidelines are listed here: www.avon company.com/women/avonfoundation/gapeop.html.

Specific Ways to Partner

- **Coordinate on Grants:** While NBCCEDP programs are not eligible for direct grant funding from Avon BHOP, you can work with the Foundation grantees to jointly conduct targeted outreach and recruitment, and then provide preventive screenings to program-eligible women identified through that outreach. To see a full list of what organizations are currently funded by the Foundation grants, visit: www.avonbreastcare.org/fundingprograms.htm. NBCCEDP programs can also encourage qualifying organizations to apply for the Foundation grants, and then coordinate with them to provide screenings if they are awarded funding. This is particularly important if there is a waiting list for screening through your program. Information about applying for grants is available at www. avonbreastcare.org. Requests for proposals are posted annually in July. *For more information about partnering with Avon BHOP grantees, please contact The Avon Foundation Breast Care Fund Coordinating Center at info@cicatelli.org.*

- **Communicate Openly and Share Information:** Your program is encouraged to communicate with the Foundation's five regional liaisons across the U.S. You can also voice your community's particular needs, as it may be possible for Avon to use this information to inform which community-based organizations are funded annually.

- **Share Resources:** NBCCEDP programs and the Foundation can share data and statistics, materials, and marketing/promotion resources. This data can help show the need in specific areas.

Engaging, Building, Expanding: An NBCCEDP Partnership Development Toolkit
Partnership Development Resources: Working with Our National Partners

March 2011

2

Working with Our National Partners

- **Communicate on a Regular Basis:** NBCCEDP programs are encouraged to regularly communicate with Avon grantees and reintroduce themselves as needed to keep their partnerships strong.

- **Support the Avon Walk:** NBCCEDP programs can send program materials to Avon Walks, which are two-day walks around the country that raise funds to advance access to care and find a cure for breast cancer. Making your materials available at the annual walks in Boston, Charlotte, Chicago, Denver/Rocky Mountains, Houston, Los Angeles/Santa Barbara, New York, San Francisco, and Washington DC can generate visibility for your program. More information is available at www.avonwalk.org. If you have an interest in sending program materials to be displayed at an Avon Walk, please contact info@avonfoundation.org.

For more information about the Avon Foundation for Women, go to www.avonfoundation.org.

Susan G. Komen for the Cure®

Susan G. Komen for the Cure® (Komen) is a nonprofit organization with a mission to end breast cancer forever. As the world's largest grassroots network of breast cancer survivors and activists, Komen receives contributions from partners, sponsors, and fellow supporters to reach millions of people and raise money for breast cancer research, education, screening, and treatment. Komen has invested nearly $1.5 billion to fulfill its promise, becoming the world's largest source of nonprofit funds dedicated to the fight against breast cancer.

The Komen Affiliate Network (the Network) consists of more than 120 local affiliates across the country. Komen affiliates raise money through Komen Race for the Cure® and other events, and 75% of the funds raised remain in the local communities to support breast cancer education, screening and treatment projects. NBCCEDP programs are encouraged to develop relationships and collaborate with the affiliates in their regions. A list of affiliates can be accessed online at http://ww5.komen.org/affiliates.aspx. Many affiliates have their own web sites that can be referenced for additional information.

The Komen Advocacy Alliance is the nonpartisan voice of the 2.5 million breast cancer survivors and the people who love them. Its mission is to ensure that its promise to save lives and end breast cancer is fulfilled through actions at all levels of government to discover and deliver the cures. The Komen Advocacy Alliance educates both federal and state legislators about NBCCEDP and actively advocates for program funding.

Specific Ways to Partner

- **Apply for Grants from the Komen Affiliate Network:** In the last five years, the Network has awarded more than $160 million in need-based community grants for breast health education and breast cancer screening programs. NBCCEDP programs are encouraged to contact local Komen affiliates to learn about available grants.

- **Provide Information and Input for Community Profiles:** In order to ensure they are funding programs that address the specific unmet breast health needs of their communities, Komen affiliates work with local medical experts and community leaders to conduct comprehensive community needs assessments. These community profiles are then used to establish local grant application and review processes consistent with Komen's standards and mission. NBCCEDP programs are encouraged to partner with Komen affiliates to provide input and data for the community profile to help ensure that Komen Affiliate grants support and supplement NBCCEDP's efforts.

- **Provide Screening Services:** Your program can screen women identified through Komen's grassroots efforts, which may include targeted outreach and recruitment for NBCCEDP among priority populations.

Engaging, Building, Expanding: An NBCCEDP Partnership Development Toolkit
Partnership Development Resources: Working with Our National Partners

March 2011

3

Working with Our National Partners

- **Support Advocacy Efforts:** Provide local data and statistics to aid in the Komen Advocacy Alliance's efforts with legislators to expand local program funding. NBCCEDP programs are encouraged to share anecdotal or quantitative evidence of how projects funded by Komen have positively affected the lives of women. You can also sign up for action alerts online at www.komenadvocacy.org to find out about local advocacy-related activities in which you can get involved.

- **Utilize Professional Development Resources:** Many Komen affiliates offer tools, training and technical assistance to potential grantees. Grant writing workshops are offered to potential grantees, including NBCCEDP programs, to ensure that applicants understand the proper way to request funds and grants. If offered in your area, Komen encourages your attendance at these grant writing sessions. To learn what resources are available in your area, please contact your local affiliate.

- **Jointly Conduct Outreach to Health Care Providers:** To ensure that health care providers are encouraging mammograms for early detection of breast cancer, NBCCEDP programs and Komen can pool resources to create and send a direct mail piece reminding them of the importance of early detection. They can also collaborate on recruiting providers through outreach to professional organizations whose members include health care providers.

- **Collaborate through Local Coalitions and Advisory Boards:** NBCCEDP programs can lead or participate in coalitions or advisory boards, which may include Komen affiliates, bringing together a range of people with diverse skill sets and areas of expertise. Collaboration facilitates open discussions about how to collectively solve problems related to issues such as shortages or other concerns.

- **Communicate on a Regular Basis:** As with other nonprofit organizations, turnover can be high at affiliate chapters. NBCCEDP programs are encouraged to regularly communicate with affiliates and reintroduce themselves as needed to keep their partnerships strong.

For more information about partnering with Susan G. Komen for the Cure®, please visit www.Komen.org.

Engaging, Building, Expanding: An NBCCEDP Partnership Development Toolkit
Partnership Development Resources: Working with Our National Partners

March 2011

4

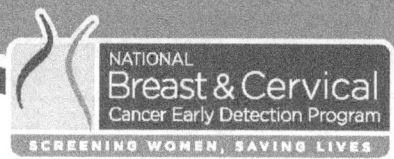

Sample Elevator Speech

Imagine you are alone in an elevator with the head of the largest employer in your area. In the short time it takes you to arrive at the lobby, what do you say? Could you readily describe your program and the benefits of partnering? This kind of "elevator speech" can be useful for delivering a concise yet complete message. The sample elevator speech below can serve as a starting point for making your own. Tailor the speech to your particular audience and what you are trying to accomplish.

TIP: Practice your speech, but don't try to memorize it word-for-word.
Relying on memory can cause you to freeze up.

SAMPLE ELEVATOR SPEECH

Did you know that nearly 45,000 women in the U.S. die from breast and cervical cancers combined each year? Fortunately, both breast and cervical cancers are treatable when found early through regular screenings. My program, **[PROGRAM NAME]**, a grant recipient of CDC's National Breast and Cervical Cancer Early Detection Program, provides regular screenings for underserved women in **[COMMUNITY NAME]**, for free or at a minimal cost. Our services help protect women in the prime of their lives, allowing them to maintain productivity and continue as primary caregivers for their families.

With more women in need of services than in years past, we need greater resources now, more than ever before. We are currently looking for support from organizations—like yours—to provide monetary or in-kind donations to help our program continue serving women in our community. Any contribution can help make a difference. Among other benefits of being a program partner, your organization can raise its visibility as a caring member of the community.

CUSTOMIZE YOUR MESSAGE

Add emotional appeal by including detailed information about the women in your community or state, the "costs" of missed screenings, and your program's impact on saving women's lives.

Think about what your program can specifically benefit from (e.g., financial vs. in-kind support) and tailor the speech to include that. If you know how many women can be screened with $1,000, or some other monetary amount, provide that information.

Add specific benefits of being a partner of your program, such as any state tax benefits.

Engaging, Building, Expanding: An NBCCEDP Partnership Development Toolkit
Partnership Development Resources: Sample Elevator Speech

March 2011

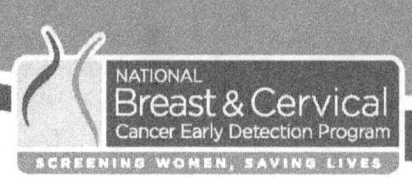

Sample Pitch Letter

The pitch letter is an important tool for introducing your program to a potential partner and starting a conversation about possible partnership opportunities. To craft the letter, make sure to research the background and goals of the organization. Think about questions like: Do they have a strong female employee or customer base? What groups have they worked with before? How can your work together be mutually beneficial? The following sample pitch letter can serve as a base for developing your own pitch. Tailor the letter to your particular audience and what you are trying to accomplish.

SAMPLE PITCH LETTER

Dear **[NAME]**,

Each year, nearly 45,000 women in the United States die from breast and cervical cancers combined, and treatment for these cancers costs more than $10 billion. The good news is that both breast and cervical cancer are treatable when found early through regular screenings. For the past 20 years, the federally funded National Breast and Cervical Cancer Early Detection Program (NBCCEDP) has been working to fight against these cancers by providing services to more than 3.7 million low-income, uninsured, and underserved women through its 68 programs.[1]

In order to continue these efforts, we need your help. As a program of NBCCEDP, **[PROGRAM NAME]** provides consumer education, outreach, and free and low-cost breast and cervical cancer screenings and diagnostic services to women in need. Last year alone, we served **[NUMBER]** of **[COMMUNITY NAME]** women. Through our services, we help protect women in the prime of their lives, allowing them to maintain productivity and continue as primary caregivers for their families.

With more women in need of services than in years past, we need greater resources now, more than ever before. Current federal and state funding cannot fully sustain our program services. Last year we had to place **[NUMBER]** women on a waiting list because of limited resources. As a prominent member of our community, we are asking **[ORGANIZATION NAME]** for assistance in making sure we can continue to serve women in our community. With a donation of **[MONETARY AMOUNT]**, we can serve **[NUMBER]** additional women this year.

Partnering with **[PROGRAM NAME]** can benefit your organization. Working with our program ensures that your contribution will directly support women in our community—including your employees and customers in need of breast and cervical cancer screenings. Additionally, partnering with an NBCCEDP program links your organization to a credible and highly respected breast and cervical cancer program. Supporting **[PROGRAM NAME]** will enhance your organization's presence in the community, help raise your visibility as a caring corporate citizen, and heighten employee morale.

I have included a few fact sheets about our program, NBCCEDP, and the benefits of supporting the program. Truly, no contribution is too small, and we appreciate any support that you can provide.

Thank you for your consideration, and I look forward to hearing from you.

Sincerely,

[NAME]

Sample Pitch Letter

CUSTOMIZE YOUR MESSAGE

Identify the most appropriate contact to receive your pitch letter. Most organizations have community relations or partnership contacts. If a contact is not listed on its website, call the organization's main phone line and ask who oversees these areas.

Add emotional appeal by including specific information about the women in your community or state, the consequences of missed screenings, and your program's impact on saving women's lives.

Reference special populations your program serves, when relevant to the organization you are pitching.

Make a specific "ask" in your pitch. Think about your program's needs and a particular way the organization can help that is mutually beneficial. This can range from in-kind to monetary donations depending upon the need and program's ability to channel funds. Please refer to *Ways to Work With Partners* in this toolkit to generate ideas.

Reinforce specific benefits of being a program partner, such as any state tax benefits.

References

1 Centers for Disease Control and Prevention, National Breast and Cervical Cancer Early Detection Program. *Minimum Data Elements*. April 2010.

Engaging, Building, Expanding: An NBCCEDP Partnership Development Toolkit
Partnership Development Resources: Sample Pitch Letter

March 2011

2

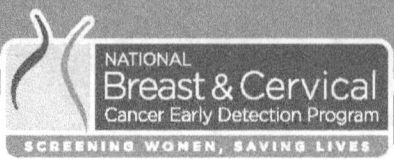

Sample Answers to Common Partner Questions

To prepare for discussions with partner prospects, think through some of the questions that you might receive during your pitch. Anticipating and being prepared to address these questions will help strengthen your case. To help get you started, below are a series of questions that you may be asked, with sample responses. Make sure to tailor responses to your program's specific situation.

Why do you need extra funds, if you already receive funding from the federal and state governments?

More women are in need of the National Breast and Cervical Cancer Early Detection Program (NBCCEDP) services than in years past, meaning we need resources now, more than ever before. Federal and state funding alone cannot fully sustain the life-saving services offered by **[PROGRAM NAME]**. Partner support is needed. If federal funding remains constant, the amount of funding received by programs each year for education and screening does not go as far due to inflation. Additionally, as an NBCCEDP program, we are required to match every $3 of federal funds that we receive with $1 of non-federal monetary or in-kind resources. While state funds count toward the matching requirements, **[STATE]** is reducing its funding due to larger budget issues.

We have a really tight budget now. Are there other ways to help?

Any contribution—no matter how big or small—is helpful. Beyond monetary partnerships, we are looking for help with **[IN-KIND PARTNERSHIP (use *Ways to Work With Partners* in this toolkit for ideas)]**. This will help us **[ACTIVITY/GOAL (e.g., staff events, drive priority populations, fund community education or extra screenings)]** and continue to serve women in our community.

Is your program community-based? We prefer to work with national programs that are highly visible and have established reputations.

Working with **[PROGRAM NAME]** connects your organization with the Centers for Disease Control and Prevention's (CDC) NBCCEDP—a respected national program that has served more than 3.7 million women and provided more than 9.2 million screening examinations over the past 20 years.[1] A partnership with **[PROGRAM NAME]** allows organizations to connect with the national program, while providing vital, on-the-ground assistance to women in need of breast and cervical cancer services within our community.

What does it mean to partner with your program? What level of effort is involved on my end?

Being our partner means supporting the women in your community. Our partners assist in a variety of ways—from providing monetary contributions to in-kind contributions, such as consumer education, provider education, printing, translation services, recruitment, fundraising, meeting facility provision, and advocacy. The level of effort depends on how you can and would like to contribute—as much or as little as you would like.

Sample Answers to Common Partner Questions

What does your program do with partner resources?

Funding and in-kind contributions and support helps **[PROGRAM NAME]** provide women access to needed education, outreach, screening, and other breast and cervical cancer-related services to women in our community. By providing **[RESOURCE, e.g., funding, supplies, staff]**, we will be able to **[ACTIVITY/GOAL]**.

How does a partnership benefit my organization?

By working with **[PROGRAM NAME]**, your contribution will directly support women in our community who need breast and cervical cancer education and screenings. Supporting our program will enhance your organization's presence in the community, help raise your visibility as a caring corporate citizen, and heighten employee morale. Additionally, partnering with an NBCCEDP program provides your organization with exposure to a new audience of supporters or customers, while linking your organization with CDC's highly credible and respected breast and cervical cancer program.

Do you have data to support the impact/success/quality of your program?

In **[YEAR]**, we served **[NUMBER]** women in the area—providing **[NUMBER]** mammograms and **[NUMBER]** Pap smears. This year, we hope to serve **[NUMBER]** women, but could serve more with your help. The program is evaluated semi-annually by CDC against quality indicators. (Share *Program Profile Template* from this toolkit and any other relevant data.)

How will I know the impact of my contribution?

We rigorously evaluate our program on a yearly basis to ensure we are meeting our program's and CDC's goals. We are happy to follow up with you and share results from your contributions. For example, last year, **[ORGANIZATION]** supported us through **[DESCRIBE PARTNERSHIP (e.g., donating $1,000, placing an advertisement, volunteering staff time)]** allowing us to **[RESULT (e.g., serve [NUMBER] women, increase event attendance, reach out to special populations)]**.

References

1 Centers for Disease Control and Prevention, National Breast and Cervical Cancer Early Detection Program. *Minimum Data Elements.* April 2010.

Engaging, Building, Expanding: An NBCCEDP Partnership Development Toolkit
Partnership Development Resources: Sample Answers to Common Partner Questions

March 2011

2

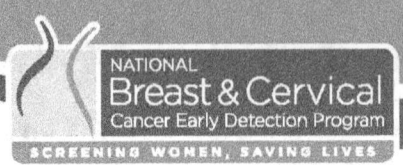

Resources

The list below includes online resources offered by the Centers for Disease Control and Prevention (CDC) and other federal agencies that can support partnership development and programmatic efforts for the National Breast and Cervical Cancer Early Detection Program (NBCCEDP) programs. These resources contain information for public education and outreach; local, state, and national statistics and data; and tools for program planning.

PUBLIC EDUCATION

- **NBCCEDP**
  Provides an overview of NBCCEDP, including: history, screening data, program highlights, and training materials. **www.cdc.gov/cancer/nbccedp/**

- **NBCCEDP Resources**
  Contains resources for NBCCEDP programs, including: data resources, information on Minimum Data Elements (MDEs), current news, meetings, and past *Ask Dr. Miller* newsletters. **www.nbccedp.org**

- *Inside Knowledge* **campaign**
  Website for *Inside Knowledge* campaign established to raise awareness of the five main types of gynecologic cancer: cervical, ovarian, uterine, vaginal, and vulvar. Provides resources, consumer materials, and messages. **www.cdc.gov/cancer/knowledge/**

- **Breast Cancer**
  Comprehensive compilation of resources about breast cancer, including basic facts, interactive tools, research, news, and more. Includes some nongovernment resources.
  www.nlm.nih.gov/medlineplus/breastcancer.html

- **Cervical Cancer**
  Comprehensive compilation of resources about cervical cancer, including basic facts, human papilloma-virus (HPV) information, interactive tools, and more. Includes some nongovernment resources.
  www.nlm.nih.gov/medlineplus/cervicalcancer.html

STATISTICS AND DATA

- **Behavioral Risk Factor Surveillance System (BRFSS)**
  State-based system of ongoing telephone health surveys that collects information on health risk behaviors, preventive health practices, and health care access primarily related to chronic disease and injury. Many states use BRFSS data to support health-related legislative efforts. **www.cdc.gov/brfss/**

- **CDC Wonder**
  An easy-to-use, menu-driven system that makes the information resources of the CDC available to public health professionals and the public at large. CDC Wonder provides access to a wide array of public health information, including cancer incidence and mortality data. It is also valuable in public health research, decision making, priority setting, program evaluation, and resource allocation. **http://wonder.cdc.gov/**

1

Resources

- **Current Population Survey (CPS)**
  Monthly survey of about 50,000 households conducted by the Bureau of the Census for the Bureau of Labor Statistics. The CPS is the primary source of information on the labor force characteristics of the U.S. population and can be used to estimate the number of women eligible for NBCCEDP's services in a particular area. Employment, unemployment, earnings, hours of work, and other indicators are evaluated. **www.census.gov/cps/**

- **Geographic Information Systems (GIS)**
  Mapping software allowing users to map a variable or variables by geographic area. Maps can be overlaid to show bivariate distributions, helping to visualize areas of interest. For example, GIS can depict areas in a state with high cancer mortality rates and then overlay those with locations of screening providers—which can inform how NBCCEDP resources can most efficiently be utilized. **http://gis.cancer.gov/**

- **Interactive Cancer Atlas (InCA)**
  Allows users to create customized United States maps showing how many people were diagnosed with or died from cancer by cancer site, gender, race/ethnicity, and state during a given period. InCA uses data from United States Cancer Statistics (USCS), the official federal statistics on cancer incidence. **http://www.cdc.gov/Features/CancerAtlas/**

- **Morbidity and Mortality Weekly Report State Health Statistics**
  Based on weekly reports to CDC by state health departments. The reporting week concludes at close of business on Friday, and compiled data on a national basis are officially released to the public on the following Friday. **www.cdc.gov/mmwr/StateHealth/index.html**

- **National Program of Cancer Registries**
  Data collected by local cancer registries to help enable public health professionals to understand and address the cancer burden more effectively. Data includes: occurrence of cancer; the type, extent, and location of the cancer; and the type of initial treatment related to cancer cases and deaths in the U.S. **www.cdc.gov/cancer/npcr/**

- **Surveillance, Epidemiology and End Results (SEER) Cancer Statistics**
  Collects information on incidence, prevalence, and survival from specific geographic areas representing 26% of the U.S. population. Compiles reports on all of these plus cancer mortality for the entire country. **http://seer.cancer.gov/**

- **State Cancer Profiles**
  Comprehensive system of interactive maps and graphs enabling the investigation of cancer trends at the national, state, and county levels. Aims to provide a system to characterize the cancer burden in a standardized manner in order to motivate action, integrate surveillance into cancer control planning, characterize areas and demographic groups, and expose health disparities. It is a collaboration between the National Cancer Institute (NCI) and CDC. **http://statecancerprofiles.cancer.gov/**

- **U.S. Cancer Statistics**
  Contains the official federal statistics on cancer incidence (newly diagnosed cases) from each registry that met data quality criteria. CDC and NCI have combined their cancer incidence data sources to produce these statistics. Mortality data from CDC's National Vital Statistics System are also included for each state. **http://apps.nccd.cdc.gov/uscs/**

Resources

PROGRAM PLANNING

- **Cancer Control P.L.A.N.E.T.**
  Portal providing access to data and resources that can help planners, program staff, and researchers to design, implement, and evaluate evidence-based cancer control programs.
  http://cancercontrolplanet.cancer.gov/

- **Guide to Community Preventive Services**
  Free resource to help program planners choose programs and policies to improve health and prevent disease in their communities. More than 200 interventions have been reviewed, and the Task Force on Community Preventive Services has issued recommendations for their use.
  http://thecommunityguide.org/index.html

- **National Comprehensive Cancer Control Program (NCCCP)**
  Established in 1998 by CDC, provides seed money and technical support for the development and implementation of plans for comprehensive cancer control, a collaborative process through which a community and its partners pool resources to reduce the burden of cancer. Like NBCCEDP, NCCCP has a national presence, with programs in all 50 states, the District of Columbia, seven tribes and tribal organizations, and seven U.S. territories. **www.cdc.gov/cancer/ncccp/**

Engaging, Building, Expanding: An NBCCEDP Partnership Development Toolkit
Partnership Development Resources: Resources

March 2011

3

About the Program

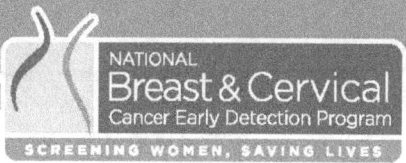

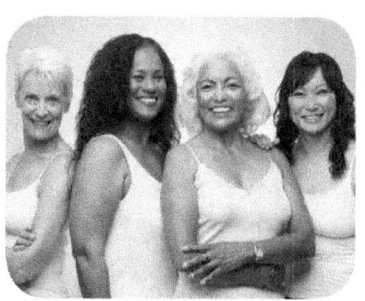

The Centers for Disease Control and Prevention's (CDC) National Breast and Cervical Cancer Early Detection Program (NBCCEDP) provides public education, free and low-cost breast and cervical cancer screenings, and diagnostic services to low-income, uninsured, and underserved women.

The National Program

To aid in the fight against breast and cervical cancer, Congress passed the Breast and Cervical Cancer Mortality Prevention Act of 1990, which guided CDC in creating NBCCEDP. In 2009, NBCCEDP provided $186 million in funding to all 50 states, the District of Columbia, five U.S. territories, and 12 American Indian/Alaska Native tribes or tribal organizations. Services included in the program are:

- Public education
- Clinical breast examinations
- Mammograms
- Pap tests
- Pelvic examinations
- Diagnostic testing, if results are abnormal
- Referrals to treatment

In 2000, Congress passed the Breast and Cervical Cancer Prevention and Treatment Act to give states the option of offering women in NBCCEDP access to treatment through a special Medicaid option program. All 50 states and the District of Columbia have approved this Medicaid option. In 2001, passage of the Native American Breast and Cervical Cancer Treatment Technical Amendment Act by Congress expanded this option to provide access to treatment to American Indians and Alaska Natives through the Indian Health Service or a tribal organization.

Program Eligibility

Federal guidelines establish eligibility to uninsured and underinsured women at or below 250% of federal poverty level, ages 40-64 for breast cancer screening, and 18-64 for cervical cancer screening. An estimated 8%-11% of U.S. women of screening age are eligible to receive NBCCEDP services.

The Burden of Breast and Cervical Cancer

Breast and cervical cancers claim the lives of thousands of women each year. Breast cancer is the second most commonly diagnosed cancer among women in the United States (after skin cancer) and the second most common cause of cancer death (after lung cancer) among U.S. women.[1] Each year, approximately 190,000 women are diagnosed with breast cancer and 40,000 women die from the disease.[1] More than $8.1 billion per year (in 2004 dollars) is spent in the United States on the treatment of breast cancer.[2]

About the Program

Cervical cancer was once the leading cause of death for women in the United States. However, during the past 50 years, incidence (the number of new cases each year) and mortality (the number of deaths each year) from cervical cancer have declined 75%, largely because of the widespread use of the Papanicolaou (Pap) test to detect cervical abnormalities.[3] Each year, approximately 12,000 women are diagnosed with cervical cancer and 4,000 women die from the disease.[1] It is estimated that more than $2 billion (in 2000 dollars) is spent on the treatment of cervical cancer per year in the U.S.[4]

The Benefits of Screening

Mammography is the best available method to detect breast cancer in its earliest, most treatable form. Studies show that early detection of breast cancer can save lives. Mammography, performed every one to two years for women aged 40 years or older, can reduce mortality by approximately 20%–25% over 10 years.[5]

Cervical cancer is highly preventable if precancerous changes are identified, and it is highly treatable if cancer is detected early. Regular Pap tests decrease a woman's risk of developing cervical cancer by detecting precancerous cervical lesions, which can be treated effectively.[3]

If screening rates among women at risk increased, deaths from breast and cervical cancers could be avoided. Deaths from these diseases occur disproportionately among women who are uninsured or underinsured. Mammography and Pap tests are underused by women who have no source or no regular source of health care, women without health insurance, and women who immigrated to the United States within the past 10 years.[6]

Accomplishments

Since 1991, NBCCEDP programs have served more than 3.7 million women, and provided more than 9.2 million breast and cervical cancer screening examinations.[7] In program year 2009, the NBCCEDP:

- Screened 324,912 women for breast cancer with mammography and found 4,635 breast cancers.
- Screened 320,627 women for cervical cancer with the Pap test and found 4,694 cervical cancers and high-grade precancerous lesions.

Program Outlook:
The Value of Partnerships

Federal funding alone cannot fully sustain NBCCEDP programs. While NBCCEDP programs maximize available funding for their services, the current level of funding only supports screening for 15.9% of eligible women for breast cancer and 8.7% of eligible women for cervical cancer. Partners are needed to provide a range of in-kind and monetary contributions to help programs provide greater access to critically needed breast and cervical cancer-related services.

References

1 U.S. Cancer Statistics Working Group. United States Cancer Statistics: 1999 2006 Incidence and Mortality Web based Report. Atlanta, GA: Department of Health and Human Services, Centers for Disease Control and Prevention, and National Cancer Institute; 2010. Available at: http://www.cdc.gov/uscs.

2 National Cancer Institute. Cancer Trends Progress Report 2007 Update. Bethesda, MD: U.S. Department of Health and Human Services, National Institutes of Health. Available at http://progressreport.cancer.gov. In 2004 dollars, based on methods described in Medical Care 2002;40(8 Suppl):IV 104 117.

3 National Institutes of Health. Cervical Cancer. NIH Consensus Statement. 1996;14(1):1 38.

4 Brown ML, Lipscomb J, Snyder C. The burden of illness of cancer: economic cost and quality of life. Annual Review of Public Health 2001; 22:91 113.

5 U.S. Preventive Services Task Force. What's New from the U.S. Preventive Services Task Force? Screening for Breast Cancer. Rockville, MD: Agency for Healthcare Research and Quality; 2002.

6 Pleis JR, Schiller JS, Benson V. Summary health statistics for U.S. adults: National Health Interview Survey, 2000. Vital and Health Statistics. Series 10, Data from the National Health Survey. 2003; (215):1 132.

7 Centers for Disease Control and Prevention, National Breast and Cervical Cancer Early Detection Program. Minimum Data Elements. April 2010.

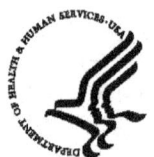 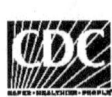

Centers for Disease Control and Prevention
National Breast and Cervical Cancer
Early Detection Program
1 (800) CDC INFO • CDCINFO@cdc.gov
www.cdc.gov/cancer/nbccedp/

About the Program

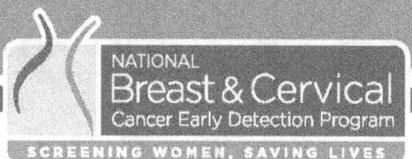

NATIONAL
Breast & Cervical
Cancer Early Detection Program
SCREENING WOMEN, SAVING LIVES

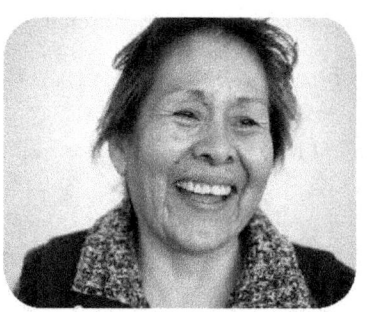

The Centers for Disease Control and Prevention's (CDC) National Breast and Cervical Cancer Early Detection Program (NBCCEDP) provides public education, free and low-cost breast and cervical cancer screenings, and diagnostic services to low-income, uninsured, and underserved women.

The National Program

To aid in the fight against breast and cervical cancer, Congress passed the Breast and Cervical Cancer Mortality Prevention Act of 1990, which guided CDC in creating NBCCEDP. In 2009, NBCCEDP provided $186 million in funding to all 50 states, the District of Columbia, five U.S. territories, and 12 American Indian/Alaska Native tribes or tribal organizations. Services included in the program are:

- Public education
- Clinical breast examinations
- Mammograms
- Pap tests
- Pelvic examinations
- Diagnostic testing, if results are abnormal
- Referrals to treatment

In 2000, Congress passed the Breast and Cervical Cancer Prevention and Treatment Act to give states the option of offering women in NBCCEDP access to treatment through a special Medicaid option program. All 50 states and the District of Columbia have approved this Medicaid option. In 2001, passage of the Native American Breast and Cervical Cancer Treatment Technical Amendment Act by Congress expanded this option to provide access to treatment to American Indians and Alaska Natives through the Indian Health Service or a tribal organization.

Program Eligibility

Federal guidelines establish eligibility to uninsured and underinsured women at or below 250% of federal poverty level, ages 40-64 for breast cancer screening, and 18-64 for cervical cancer screening. An estimated 8%-11% of U.S. women of screening age are eligible to receive NBCCEDP services.

The Burden of Breast and Cervical Cancer

Breast and cervical cancers claim the lives of thousands of women each year. Breast cancer is the second most commonly diagnosed cancer among women in the United States (after skin cancer) and the second most common cause of cancer death (after lung cancer) among U.S. women.[1] Each year, approximately 190,000 women are diagnosed with breast cancer and 40,000 women die from the disease.[1] More than $8.1 billion per year (in 2004 dollars) is spent in the United States on the treatment of breast cancer.[2]

About the Program

Cervical cancer was once the leading cause of death for women in the United States. However, during the past 50 years, incidence (the number of new cases each year) and mortality (the number of deaths each year) from cervical cancer have declined 75%, largely because of the widespread use of the Papanicolaou (Pap) test to detect cervical abnormalities.[3] Each year, approximately 12,000 women are diagnosed with cervical cancer and 4,000 women die from the disease.[1] It is estimated that more than $2 billion (in 2000 dollars) is spent on the treatment of cervical cancer per year in the U.S.[4]

The Benefits of Screening

Mammography is the best available method to detect breast cancer in its earliest, most treatable form. Studies show that early detection of breast cancer can save lives. Mammography, performed every one to two years for women aged 40 years or older, can reduce mortality by approximately 20%–25% over 10 years.[5]

Cervical cancer is highly preventable if precancerous changes are identified, and it is highly treatable if cancer is detected early. Regular Pap tests decrease a woman's risk of developing cervical cancer by detecting precancerous cervical lesions, which can be treated effectively.[3]

If screening rates among women at risk increased, deaths from breast and cervical cancers could be avoided. Deaths from these diseases occur disproportionately among women who are uninsured or underinsured. Mammography and Pap tests are underused by women who have no source or no regular source of health care, women without health insurance, and women who immigrated to the United States within the past 10 years.[6]

Accomplishments

Since 1991, NBCCEDP programs have served more than 3.7 million women, and provided more than 9.2 million breast and cervical cancer screening examinations.[7] In program year 2009, the NBCCEDP:

- Screened 324,912 women for breast cancer with mammography and found 4,635 breast cancers.
- Screened 320,627 women for cervical cancer with the Pap test and found 4,694 cervical cancers and high-grade precancerous lesions.

Program Outlook:
The Value of Partnerships

Federal funding alone cannot fully sustain NBCCEDP programs. While NBCCEDP programs maximize available funding for their services, the current level of funding only supports screening for 15.9% of eligible women for breast cancer and 8.7% of eligible women for cervical cancer. Partners are needed to provide a range of in-kind and monetary contributions to help programs provide greater access to critically needed breast and cervical cancer-related services.

References

1 U.S. Cancer Statistics Working Group. United States Cancer Statistics: 1999 2006 Incidence and Mortality Web based Report. Atlanta, GA: Department of Health and Human Services, Centers for Disease Control and Prevention, and National Cancer Institute; 2010. Available at: http://www.cdc.gov/uscs.

2 National Cancer Institute. Cancer Trends Progress Report 2007 Update. Bethesda, MD: U.S. Department of Health and Human Services, National Institutes of Health. Available at http://progressreport.cancer.gov. In 2004 dollars, based on methods described in Medical Care 2002;40(8 Suppl):IV 104 117.

3 National Institutes of Health. Cervical Cancer. NIH Consensus Statement. 1996;14(1):1 38.

4 Brown ML, Lipscomb J, Snyder C. The burden of illness of cancer: economic cost and quality of life. Annual Review of Public Health 2001; 22:91 113.

5 U.S. Preventive Services Task Force. What's New from the U.S. Preventive Services Task Force? Screening for Breast Cancer. Rockville, MD: Agency for Healthcare Research and Quality; 2002.

6 Pleis JR, Schiller JS, Benson V. Summary health statistics for U.S. adults: National Health Interview Survey, 2000. Vital and Health Statistics. Series 10, Data from the National Health Survey. 2003; (215):1 132.

7 Centers for Disease Control and Prevention, National Breast and Cervical Cancer Early Detection Program. Minimum Data Elements. April 2010.

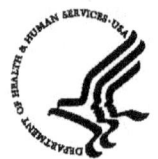 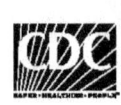

Centers for Disease Control and Prevention
National Breast and Cervical Cancer
Early Detection Program
1 (800) CDC INFO • CDCINFO@cdc.gov
www.cdc.gov/cancer/nbccedp/

About the Program

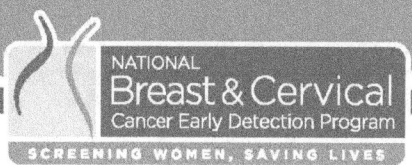

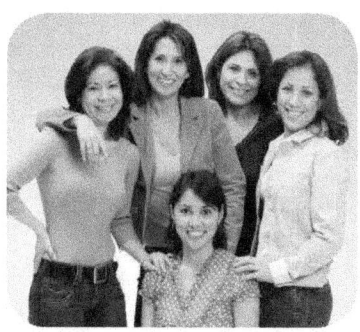

The Centers for Disease Control and Prevention's (CDC) National Breast and Cervical Cancer Early Detection Program (NBCCEDP) provides public education, free and low-cost breast and cervical cancer screenings, and diagnostic services to low-income, uninsured, and underserved women.

The National Program

To aid in the fight against breast and cervical cancer, Congress passed the Breast and Cervical Cancer Mortality Prevention Act of 1990, which guided CDC in creating NBCCEDP. In 2009, NBCCEDP provided $186 million in funding to all 50 states, the District of Columbia, five U.S. territories, and 12 American Indian/Alaska Native tribes or tribal organizations. Services included in the program are:

- Public education
- Clinical breast examinations
- Mammograms
- Pap tests
- Pelvic examinations
- Diagnostic testing, if results are abnormal
- Referrals to treatment

In 2000, Congress passed the Breast and Cervical Cancer Prevention and Treatment Act to give states the option of offering women in NBCCEDP access to treatment through a special Medicaid option program. All 50 states and the District of Columbia have approved this Medicaid option. In 2001, passage of the Native American Breast and Cervical Cancer Treatment Technical Amendment Act by Congress expanded this option to provide access to treatment to American Indians and Alaska Natives through the Indian Health Service or a tribal organization.

Program Eligibility

Federal guidelines establish eligibility to uninsured and underinsured women at or below 250% of federal poverty level, ages 40–64 for breast cancer screening, and 18–64 for cervical cancer screening. An estimated 8%–11% of U.S. women of screening age are eligible to receive NBCCEDP services.

The Burden of Breast and Cervical Cancer

Breast and cervical cancers claim the lives of thousands of women each year. Breast cancer is the second most commonly diagnosed cancer among women in the United States (after skin cancer) and the second most common cause of cancer death (after lung cancer) among U.S. women.[1] Each year, approximately 190,000 women are diagnosed with breast cancer and 40,000 women die from the disease.[1] More than $8.1 billion per year (in 2004 dollars) is spent in the United States on the treatment of breast cancer.[2]

About the Program

Cervical cancer was once the leading cause of death for women in the United States. However, during the past 50 years, incidence (the number of new cases each year) and mortality (the number of deaths each year) from cervical cancer have declined 75%, largely because of the widespread use of the Papanicolaou (Pap) test to detect cervical abnormalities.[3] Each year, approximately 12,000 women are diagnosed with cervical cancer and 4,000 women die from the disease.[1] It is estimated that more than $2 billion (in 2000 dollars) is spent on the treatment of cervical cancer per year in the U.S.[4]

The Benefits of Screening

Mammography is the best available method to detect breast cancer in its earliest, most treatable form. Studies show that early detection of breast cancer can save lives. Mammography, performed every one to two years for women aged 40 years or older, can reduce mortality by approximately 20%–25% over 10 years.[5]

Cervical cancer is highly preventable if precancerous changes are identified, and it is highly treatable if cancer is detected early. Regular Pap tests decrease a woman's risk of developing cervical cancer by detecting precancerous cervical lesions, which can be treated effectively.[3]

If screening rates among women at risk increased, deaths from breast and cervical cancers could be avoided. Deaths from these diseases occur disproportionately among women who are uninsured or underinsured. Mammography and Pap tests are underused by women who have no source or no regular source of health care, women without health insurance, and women who immigrated to the United States within the past 10 years.[6]

Accomplishments

Since 1991, NBCCEDP programs have served more than 3.7 million women, and provided more than 9.2 million breast and cervical cancer screening examinations.[7] In program year 2009, the NBCCEDP:

- Screened 324,912 women for breast cancer with mammography and found 4,635 breast cancers.
- Screened 320,627 women for cervical cancer with the Pap test and found 4,694 cervical cancers and high-grade precancerous lesions.

Program Outlook: The Value of Partnerships

Federal funding alone cannot fully sustain NBCCEDP programs. While NBCCEDP programs maximize available funding for their services, the current level of funding only supports screening for 15.9% of eligible women for breast cancer and 8.7% of eligible women for cervical cancer. Partners are needed to provide a range of in-kind and monetary contributions to help programs provide greater access to critically needed breast and cervical cancer-related services.

References

1 U.S. Cancer Statistics Working Group. United States Cancer Statistics: 1999 2006 Incidence and Mortality Web based Report. Atlanta, GA: Department of Health and Human Services, Centers for Disease Control and Prevention, and National Cancer Institute; 2010. Available at: http://www.cdc.gov/uscs.

2 National Cancer Institute. Cancer Trends Progress Report 2007 Update. Bethesda, MD: U.S. Department of Health and Human Services, National Institutes of Health. Available at http://progressreport.cancer.gov. In 2004 dollars, based on methods described in Medical Care 2002;40(8 Suppl):IV 104 117.

3 National Institutes of Health. Cervical Cancer. NIH Consensus Statement. 1996;14(1):1 38.

4 Brown ML, Lipscomb J, Snyder C. The burden of illness of cancer: economic cost and quality of life. Annual Review of Public Health 2001; 22:91 113.

5 U.S. Preventive Services Task Force. What's New from the U.S. Preventive Services Task Force? Screening for Breast Cancer. Rockville, MD: Agency for Healthcare Research and Quality; 2002.

6 Pleis JR, Schiller JS, Benson V. Summary health statistics for U S. adults: National Health Interview Survey, 2000. Vital and Health Statistics. Series 10, Data from the National Health Survey. 2003; (215):1 132.

7 Centers for Disease Control and Prevention, National Breast and Cervical Cancer Early Detection Program. Minimum Data Elements. April 2010.

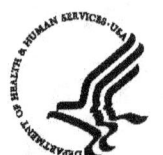 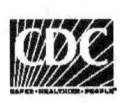

Centers for Disease Control and Prevention
National Breast and Cervical Cancer
Early Detection Program
1 (800) CDC INFO • CDCINFO@cdc.gov
www.cdc.gov/cancer/nbccedp/

Breast Cancer Facts

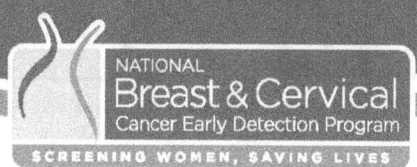

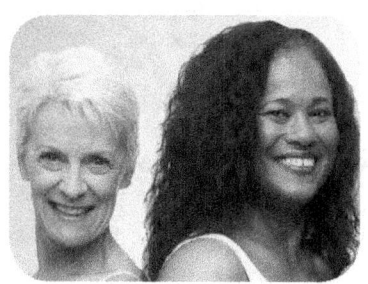

Breast Cancer

Breast cancer claims the lives of thousands of women in the United States each year. Learn basic information about breast cancer and how to prevent and recognize it.

What is breast cancer?

Cancer is a disease in which cells in the body grow out of control. When cancer starts in the breast, it is called breast cancer. The breast is made up of three main parts: glands, ducts, and connective tissue. Sometimes, breast cells become abnormal and grow faster than normal cells. These extra cells form a mass called a tumor. Some tumors are "benign," or not cancerous. Other tumors are "malignant," meaning they are cancerous and have the ability to spread to other parts of the breast and body and disrupt normal functions in those areas.

All women are at risk for breast cancer. Men can also get breast cancer, but this is rare. Breast cancer is the second most common cancer in women. Among Hispanic women, it is the most common cause of cancer deaths, and it is the second most common cause of cancer deaths among white, black, Asian or Pacific Islander, and American Indian or Alaska Native women. Although more white women get breast cancer, more black women die from it. Each year, approximately 190,000 women are diagnosed with breast cancer and 40,000 women die from the disease.[1]

What puts me at greater risk?

Several factors may affect your risk of developing breast cancer, including:

* Getting older
* Not having children, or having your first child later in life
* Starting your first menstrual period at an early age
* Beginning menopause at a late age
* Having a personal history of breast cancer or certain benign breast diseases, such as atypical ductal hyperplasia
* Having close family relatives (such as a mother, sister, father, or daughter) who have had breast cancer
* Having a genetic condition, such as certain mutations in your BRCA1 or BRCA2 genes
* Having been treated with radiation therapy to the breast or chest
* Being overweight, particularly after menopause
* Using hormone replacement therapy for a long time
* Using oral contraceptives
* Drinking alcohol
* Being physically inactive

Breast Cancer Facts

What are the symptoms?

When breast cancer starts out, it is too small to feel and does not cause signs and symptoms. As it grows, however, breast cancer can cause changes in how the breast looks or feels. Symptoms may include:

- A new lump in the breast
- A lump that has changed
- A change in the size or shape of the breast
- Pain in the breast or nipple that does not go away
- Flaky, red, or swollen skin anywhere on the breast
- A nipple that is very tender or that turns inward
- Blood or any other type of fluid coming from the nipple that is not milk when nursing a baby

These symptoms may be caused by something other than cancer, but the only way to know is to get checked.

How can I find out if I have breast cancer?

Women should begin to have routine screenings for breast cancer at the age of 50. Women under the age of 50 should talk to their health care provider about when and how often they should be screened.

If you have any risk factors or symptoms of breast cancer, talk to a doctor, nurse, or health care professional.

A mammogram is the best test for finding breast cancer early. It is a series of X-ray pictures of the breast that allow doctors to look for early signs of breast cancer, sometimes up to three years before it can be felt.

If your mammogram is abnormal or more tests are required, do not panic. An abnormal mammogram does not always mean you have cancer. It does mean that you will need to have some additional X-rays or other tests before your doctor can be sure. Other tests may include an ultrasound (picture taken of the breast using sound waves) or a biopsy (removing tissue samples to be looked at closely under a microscope). You may be referred to a breast specialist or a surgeon, because these doctors are experts in diagnosing breast problems.

Treatment is most effective when breast cancer is found early, and many women go on to live long and healthy lives.

How can I prevent breast cancer?

Scientists are studying how best to prevent breast cancer. There are things you can do to help lower your risk of getting breast cancer, including:

- Staying physically active with regular exercise
- Maintaining a healthy weight
- Avoiding hormone replacement therapy (HRT), or finding out the risks and benefits of HRT and if it is right for you
- Limiting the amount of alcohol that you drink

About the National Breast and Cervical Cancer Early Detection Program (NBCCEDP)

NBCCEDP provides public education, free and low-cost breast and cervical cancer screenings, and diagnostic services to low-income, uninsured, and underserved women. If you have a low income or do not have insurance, and are between the ages of 40 and 64, you may be able to get a free or low-cost mammogram through the NBCCEDP in your community.

References

1 U.S. Cancer Statistics Working Group. *United States Cancer Statistics: 1999 2006 Incidence and Mortality Web based Report.* Atlanta, GA: Department of Health and Human Services, Centers for Disease Control and Prevention, and National Cancer Institute; 2010. Available at: http://www.cdc.gov/uscs.

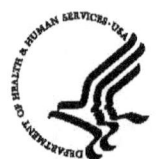 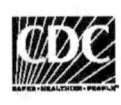

Centers for Disease Control and Prevention
National Breast and Cervical Cancer
Early Detection Program
1 (800) CDC INFO • CDCINFO@cdc.gov
www.cdc.gov/cancer/nbccedp/

Breast Cancer Facts

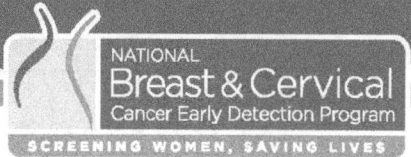

NATIONAL
Breast & Cervical
Cancer Early Detection Program
SCREENING WOMEN, SAVING LIVES

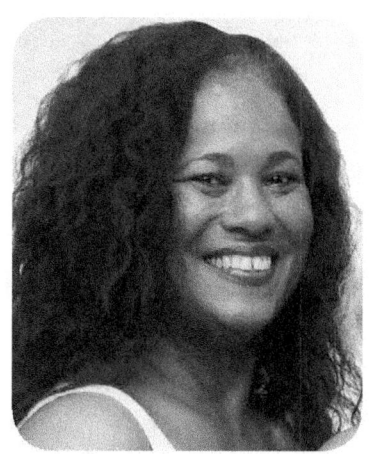

Breast Cancer

Breast cancer claims the lives of thousands of women in the United States each year. Learn basic information about breast cancer and how to prevent and recognize it.

What is breast cancer?

Cancer is a disease in which cells in the body grow out of control. When cancer starts in the breast, it is called breast cancer. The breast is made up of three main parts: glands, ducts, and connective tissue. Sometimes, breast cells become abnormal and grow faster than normal cells. These extra cells form a mass called a tumor. Some tumors are "benign," or not cancerous. Other tumors are "malignant," meaning they are cancerous and have the ability to spread to other parts of the breast and body and disrupt normal functions in those areas.

All women are at risk for breast cancer. Men can also get breast cancer, but this is rare. Breast cancer is the second most common cancer in women. Among Hispanic women, it is the most common cause of cancer deaths, and it is the second most common cause of cancer deaths among white, black, Asian or Pacific Islander, and American Indian or Alaska Native women. Although more white women get breast cancer, more black women die from it. Each year, approximately 190,000 women are diagnosed with breast cancer and 40,000 women die from the disease.[1]

What puts me at greater risk?

Several factors may affect your risk of developing breast cancer, including:

- Getting older
- Not having children, or having your first child later in life
- Starting your first menstrual period at an early age
- Beginning menopause at a late age
- Having a personal history of breast cancer or certain benign breast diseases, such as atypical ductal hyperplasia
- Having close family relatives (such as a mother, sister, father, or daughter) who have had breast cancer
- Having a genetic condition, such as certain mutations in your BRCA1 or BRCA2 genes
- Having been treated with radiation therapy to the breast or chest
- Being overweight, particularly after menopause
- Using hormone replacement therapy for a long time
- Using oral contraceptives
- Drinking alcohol
- Being physically inactive

Breast Cancer Facts

What are the symptoms?

When breast cancer starts out, it is too small to feel and does not cause signs and symptoms. As it grows, however, breast cancer can cause changes in how the breast looks or feels. Symptoms may include:

* A new lump in the breast
* A lump that has changed
* A change in the size or shape of the breast
* Pain in the breast or nipple that does not go away
* Flaky, red, or swollen skin anywhere on the breast
* A nipple that is very tender or that turns inward
* Blood or any other type of fluid coming from the nipple that is not milk when nursing a baby

These symptoms may be caused by something other than cancer, but the only way to know is to get checked.

How can I find out if I have breast cancer?

Women should begin to have routine screenings for breast cancer at the age of 50. Women under the age of 50 should talk to their health care provider about when and how often they should be screened.

If you have any risk factors or symptoms of breast cancer, talk to a doctor, nurse, or health care professional.

A mammogram is the best test for finding breast cancer early. It is a series of X-ray pictures of the breast that allow doctors to look for early signs of breast cancer, sometimes up to three years before it can be felt.

If your mammogram is abnormal or more tests are required, do not panic. An abnormal mammogram does not always mean you have cancer. It does mean that you will need to have some additional X-rays or other tests before your doctor can be sure. Other tests may include an ultrasound (picture taken of the breast using sound waves) or a biopsy (removing tissue samples to be looked at closely under a microscope). You may be referred to a breast specialist or a surgeon, because these doctors are experts in diagnosing breast problems.

Treatment is most effective when breast cancer is found early, and many women go on to live long and healthy lives.

How can I prevent breast cancer?

Scientists are studying how best to prevent breast cancer. There are things you can do to help lower your risk of getting breast cancer, including:

* Staying physically active with regular exercise
* Maintaining a healthy weight
* Avoiding hormone replacement therapy (HRT), or finding out the risks and benefits of HRT and if it is right for you
* Limiting the amount of alcohol that you drink

About the National Breast and Cervical Cancer Early Detection Program (NBCCEDP)

NBCCEDP provides public education, free and low-cost breast and cervical cancer screenings, and diagnostic services to low-income, uninsured, and underserved women. If you have a low income or do not have insurance, and are between the ages of 40 and 64, you may be able to get a free or low-cost mammogram through the NBCCEDP in your community.

References

1 U.S. Cancer Statistics Working Group. *United States Cancer Statistics: 1999 2006 Incidence and Mortality Web based Report.* Atlanta, GA: Department of Health and Human Services, Centers for Disease Control and Prevention, and National Cancer Institute; 2010. Available at: http://www.cdc.gov/uscs.

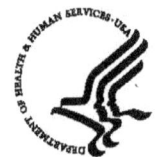 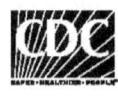

Centers for Disease Control and Prevention
National Breast and Cervical Cancer
Early Detection Program
1 (800) CDC INFO • CDCINFO@cdc.gov
www.cdc.gov/cancer/nbccedp/

Breast Cancer Facts

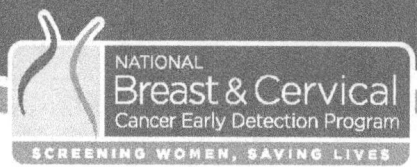

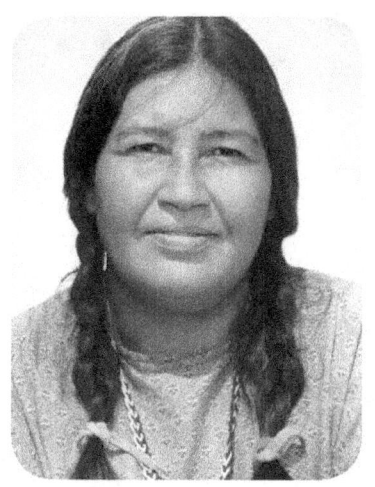

Breast Cancer

Breast cancer claims the lives of thousands of women in the United States each year. Learn basic information about breast cancer and how to prevent and recognize it.

What is breast cancer?

Cancer is a disease in which cells in the body grow out of control. When cancer starts in the breast, it is called breast cancer. The breast is made up of three main parts: glands, ducts, and connective tissue. Sometimes, breast cells become abnormal and grow faster than normal cells. These extra cells form a mass called a tumor. Some tumors are "benign," or not cancerous. Other tumors are "malignant," meaning they are cancerous and have the ability to spread to other parts of the breast and body and disrupt normal functions in those areas.

All women are at risk for breast cancer. Men can also get breast cancer, but this is rare. Breast cancer is the second most common cancer in women. Among Hispanic women, it is the most common cause of cancer deaths, and it is the second most common cause of cancer deaths among white, black, Asian or Pacific Islander, and American Indian or Alaska Native women. Although more white women get breast cancer, more black women die from it. Each year, approximately 190,000 women are diagnosed with breast cancer and 40,000 women die from the disease.[1]

What puts me at greater risk?

Several factors may affect your risk of developing breast cancer, including:

- Getting older
- Not having children, or having your first child later in life
- Starting your first menstrual period at an early age
- Beginning menopause at a late age
- Having a personal history of breast cancer or certain benign breast diseases, such as atypical ductal hyperplasia
- Having close family relatives (such as a mother, sister, father, or daughter) who have had breast cancer
- Having a genetic condition, such as certain mutations in your BRCA1 or BRCA2 genes
- Having been treated with radiation therapy to the breast or chest
- Being overweight, particularly after menopause
- Using hormone replacement therapy for a long time
- Using oral contraceptives
- Drinking alcohol
- Being physically inactive

Breast Cancer Facts

What are the symptoms?

When breast cancer starts out, it is too small to feel and does not cause signs and symptoms. As it grows, however, breast cancer can cause changes in how the breast looks or feels. Symptoms may include:

- A new lump in the breast
- A lump that has changed
- A change in the size or shape of the breast
- Pain in the breast or nipple that does not go away
- Flaky, red, or swollen skin anywhere on the breast
- A nipple that is very tender or that turns inward
- Blood or any other type of fluid coming from the nipple that is not milk when nursing a baby

These symptoms may be caused by something other than cancer, but the only way to know is to get checked.

How can I find out if I have breast cancer?

Women should begin to have routine screenings for breast cancer at the age of 50. Women under the age of 50 should talk to their health care provider about when and how often they should be screened.

If you have any risk factors or symptoms of breast cancer, talk to a doctor, nurse, or health care professional.

A mammogram is the best test for finding breast cancer early. It is a series of X-ray pictures of the breast that allow doctors to look for early signs of breast cancer, sometimes up to three years before it can be felt.

If your mammogram is abnormal or more tests are required, do not panic. An abnormal mammogram does not always mean you have cancer. It does mean that you will need to have some additional X-rays or other tests before your doctor can be sure. Other tests may include an ultrasound (picture taken of the breast using sound waves) or a biopsy (removing tissue samples to be looked at closely under a microscope). You may be referred to a breast specialist or a surgeon, because these doctors are experts in diagnosing breast problems.

Treatment is most effective when breast cancer is found early, and many women go on to live long and healthy lives.

How can I prevent breast cancer?

Scientists are studying how best to prevent breast cancer. There are things you can do to help lower your risk of getting breast cancer, including:

- Staying physically active with regular exercise
- Maintaining a healthy weight
- Avoiding hormone replacement therapy (HRT), or finding out the risks and benefits of HRT and if it is right for you
- Limiting the amount of alcohol that you drink

About the National Breast and Cervical Cancer Early Detection Program (NBCCEDP)

NBCCEDP provides public education, free and low-cost breast and cervical cancer screenings, and diagnostic services to low-income, uninsured, and underserved women. If you have a low income or do not have insurance, and are between the ages of 40 and 64, you may be able to get a free or low-cost mammogram through the NBCCEDP in your community.

References

1 U.S. Cancer Statistics Working Group. *United States Cancer Statistics: 1999 2006 Incidence and Mortality Web based Report*. Atlanta, GA: Department of Health and Human Services, Centers for Disease Control and Prevention, and National Cancer Institute; 2010. Available at: http://www.cdc.gov/uscs.

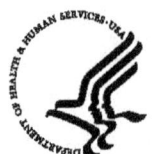 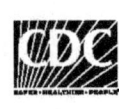

Centers for Disease Control and Prevention
National Breast and Cervical Cancer
Early Detection Program
1 (800) CDC INFO • CDCINFO@cdc.gov
www.cdc.gov/cancer/nbccedp/

Breast Cancer Facts

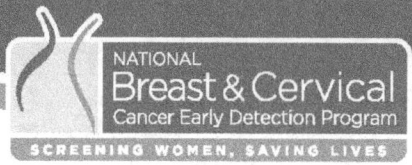

NATIONAL
Breast & Cervical
Cancer Early Detection Program
SCREENING WOMEN, SAVING LIVES

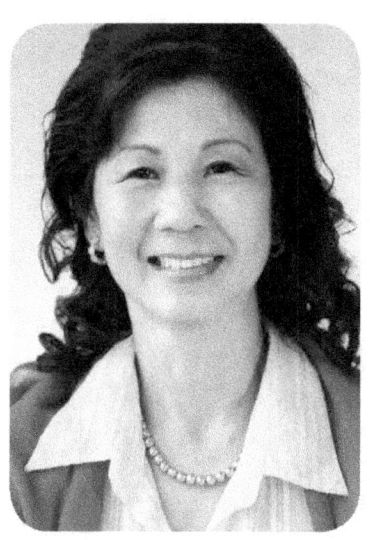

Breast Cancer

Breast cancer claims the lives of thousands of women in the United States each year. Learn basic information about breast cancer and how to prevent and recognize it.

What is breast cancer?

Cancer is a disease in which cells in the body grow out of control. When cancer starts in the breast, it is called breast cancer. The breast is made up of three main parts: glands, ducts, and connective tissue. Sometimes, breast cells become abnormal and grow faster than normal cells. These extra cells form a mass called a tumor. Some tumors are "benign," or not cancerous. Other tumors are "malignant," meaning they are cancerous and have the ability to spread to other parts of the breast and body and disrupt normal functions in those areas.

All women are at risk for breast cancer. Men can also get breast cancer, but this is rare. Breast cancer is the second most common cancer in women. Among Hispanic women, it is the most common cause of cancer deaths, and it is the second most common cause of cancer deaths among white, black, Asian or Pacific Islander, and American Indian or Alaska Native women. Although more white women get breast cancer, more black women die from it. Each year, approximately 190,000 women are diagnosed with breast cancer and 40,000 women die from the disease.[1]

What puts me at greater risk?

Several factors may affect your risk of developing breast cancer, including:

- Getting older
- Not having children, or having your first child later in life
- Starting your first menstrual period at an early age
- Beginning menopause at a late age
- Having a personal history of breast cancer or certain benign breast diseases, such as atypical ductal hyperplasia
- Having close family relatives (such as a mother, sister, father, or daughter) who have had breast cancer
- Having a genetic condition, such as certain mutations in your BRCA1 or BRCA2 genes
- Having been treated with radiation therapy to the breast or chest
- Being overweight, particularly after menopause
- Using hormone replacement therapy for a long time
- Using oral contraceptives
- Drinking alcohol
- Being physically inactive

Breast Cancer Facts

What are the symptoms?

When breast cancer starts out, it is too small to feel and does not cause signs and symptoms. As it grows, however, breast cancer can cause changes in how the breast looks or feels. Symptoms may include:

- A new lump in the breast
- A lump that has changed
- A change in the size or shape of the breast
- Pain in the breast or nipple that does not go away
- Flaky, red, or swollen skin anywhere on the breast
- A nipple that is very tender or that turns inward
- Blood or any other type of fluid coming from the nipple that is not milk when nursing a baby

These symptoms may be caused by something other than cancer, but the only way to know is to get checked.

How can I find out if I have breast cancer?

Women should begin to have routine screenings for breast cancer at the age of 50. Women under the age of 50 should talk to their health care provider about when and how often they should be screened.

If you have any risk factors or symptoms of breast cancer, talk to a doctor, nurse, or health care professional.

A mammogram is the best test for finding breast cancer early. It is a series of X-ray pictures of the breast that allow doctors to look for early signs of breast cancer, sometimes up to three years before it can be felt.

If your mammogram is abnormal or more tests are required, do not panic. An abnormal mammogram does not always mean you have cancer. It does mean that you will need to have some additional X-rays or other tests before your doctor can be sure. Other tests may include an ultrasound (picture taken of the breast using sound waves) or a biopsy (removing tissue samples to be looked at closely under a microscope). You may be referred to a breast specialist or a surgeon, because these doctors are experts in diagnosing breast problems.

Treatment is most effective when breast cancer is found early, and many women go on to live long and healthy lives.

How can I prevent breast cancer?

Scientists are studying how best to prevent breast cancer. There are things you can do to help lower your risk of getting breast cancer, including:

- Staying physically active with regular exercise
- Maintaining a healthy weight
- Avoiding hormone replacement therapy (HRT), or finding out the risks and benefits of HRT and if it is right for you
- Limiting the amount of alcohol that you drink

About the National Breast and Cervical Cancer Early Detection Program (NBCCEDP)

NBCCEDP provides public education, free and low-cost breast and cervical cancer screenings, and diagnostic services to low-income, uninsured, and underserved women. If you have a low income or do not have insurance, and are between the ages of 40 and 64, you may be able to get a free or low-cost mammogram through the NBCCEDP in your community.

References

1 U.S. Cancer Statistics Working Group. *United States Cancer Statistics: 1999 2006 Incidence and Mortality Web based Report*. Atlanta, GA: Department of Health and Human Services, Centers for Disease Control and Prevention, and National Cancer Institute; 2010. Available at: http://www.cdc.gov/uscs.

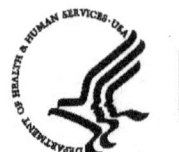 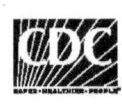

Centers for Disease Control and Prevention
National Breast and Cervical Cancer
Early Detection Program
1 (800) CDC INFO • CDCINFO@cdc.gov
www.cdc.gov/cancer/nbccedp/

Breast Cancer Facts

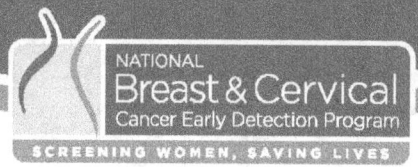

NATIONAL
Breast & Cervical
Cancer Early Detection Program
SCREENING WOMEN, SAVING LIVES

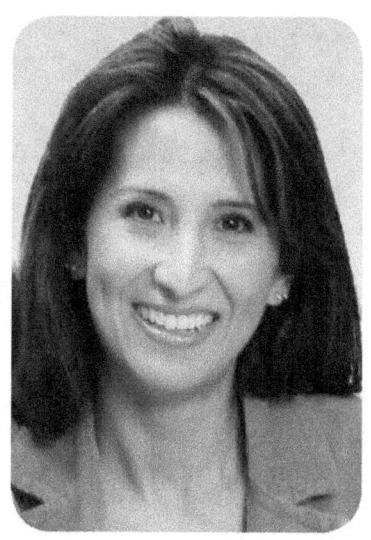

Breast Cancer

Breast cancer claims the lives of thousands of women in the United States each year. Learn basic information about breast cancer and how to prevent and recognize it.

What is breast cancer?

Cancer is a disease in which cells in the body grow out of control. When cancer starts in the breast, it is called breast cancer. The breast is made up of three main parts: glands, ducts, and connective tissue. Sometimes, breast cells become abnormal and grow faster than normal cells. These extra cells form a mass called a tumor. Some tumors are "benign," or not cancerous. Other tumors are "malignant," meaning they are cancerous and have the ability to spread to other parts of the breast and body and disrupt normal functions in those areas.

All women are at risk for breast cancer. Men can also get breast cancer, but this is rare. Breast cancer is the second most common cancer in women. Among Hispanic women, it is the most common cause of cancer deaths, and it is the second most common cause of cancer deaths among white, black, Asian or Pacific Islander, and American Indian or Alaska Native women. Although more white women get breast cancer, more black women die from it. Each year, approximately 190,000 women are diagnosed with breast cancer and 40,000 women die from the disease.[1]

What puts me at greater risk?

Several factors may affect your risk of developing breast cancer, including:

- Getting older
- Not having children, or having your first child later in life
- Starting your first menstrual period at an early age
- Beginning menopause at a late age
- Having a personal history of breast cancer or certain benign breast diseases, such as atypical ductal hyperplasia
- Having close family relatives (such as a mother, sister, father, or daughter) who have had breast cancer
- Having a genetic condition, such as certain mutations in your BRCA1 or BRCA2 genes
- Having been treated with radiation therapy to the breast or chest
- Being overweight, particularly after menopause
- Using hormone replacement therapy for a long time
- Using oral contraceptives
- Drinking alcohol
- Being physically inactive

Breast Cancer Facts

What are the symptoms?

When breast cancer starts out, it is too small to feel and does not cause signs and symptoms. As it grows, however, breast cancer can cause changes in how the breast looks or feels. Symptoms may include:

- A new lump in the breast
- A lump that has changed
- A change in the size or shape of the breast
- Pain in the breast or nipple that does not go away
- Flaky, red, or swollen skin anywhere on the breast
- A nipple that is very tender or that turns inward
- Blood or any other type of fluid coming from the nipple that is not milk when nursing a baby

These symptoms may be caused by something other than cancer, but the only way to know is to get checked.

How can I find out if I have breast cancer?

Women should begin to have routine screenings for breast cancer at the age of 50. Women under the age of 50 should talk to their health care provider about when and how often they should be screened.

If you have any risk factors or symptoms of breast cancer, talk to a doctor, nurse, or health care professional.

A mammogram is the best test for finding breast cancer early. It is a series of X-ray pictures of the breast that allow doctors to look for early signs of breast cancer, sometimes up to three years before it can be felt.

If your mammogram is abnormal or more tests are required, do not panic. An abnormal mammogram does not always mean you have cancer. It does mean that you will need to have some additional X-rays or other tests before your doctor can be sure. Other tests may include an ultrasound (picture taken of the breast using sound waves) or a biopsy (removing tissue samples to be looked at closely under a microscope). You may be referred to a breast specialist or a surgeon, because these doctors are experts in diagnosing breast problems.

Treatment is most effective when breast cancer is found early, and many women go on to live long and healthy lives.

How can I prevent breast cancer?

Scientists are studying how best to prevent breast cancer. There are things you can do to help lower your risk of getting breast cancer, including:

- Staying physically active with regular exercise
- Maintaining a healthy weight
- Avoiding hormone replacement therapy (HRT), or finding out the risks and benefits of HRT and if it is right for you
- Limiting the amount of alcohol that you drink

About the National Breast and Cervical Cancer Early Detection Program (NBCCEDP)

NBCCEDP provides public education, free and low-cost breast and cervical cancer screenings, and diagnostic services to low-income, uninsured, and underserved women. If you have a low income or do not have insurance, and are between the ages of 40 and 64, you may be able to get a free or low-cost mammogram through the NBCCEDP in your community.

References

1 U.S. Cancer Statistics Working Group. *United States Cancer Statistics: 1999 2006 Incidence and Mortality Web based Report.* Atlanta, GA: Department of Health and Human Services, Centers for Disease Control and Prevention, and National Cancer Institute; 2010. Available at: http://www.cdc.gov/uscs.

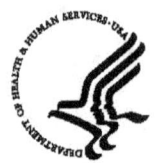 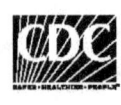

Centers for Disease Control and Prevention
National Breast and Cervical Cancer
Early Detection Program
1 (800) CDC INFO • CDCINFO@cdc.gov
www.cdc.gov/cancer/nbccedp/

Cervical Cancer Facts

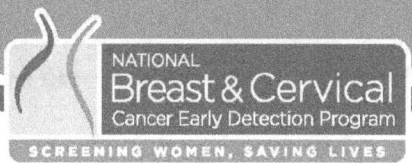

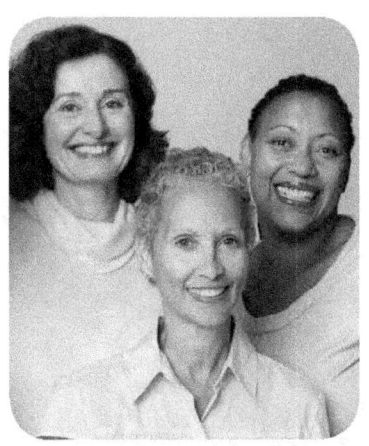

Cervical cancer is the easiest gynecological cancer to prevent with regular screening tests and follow-up. Learn basic information about cervical cancer and how to prevent and recognize it.

What is cervical cancer?

Cancer is a disease in which cells in the body grow out of control. Cancer is always named for the part of the body where it starts, even if it spreads to other body parts later. When cancer starts in the cervix, it is called cervical cancer. The cervix is the lower, narrow end of the uterus. The cervix connects the vagina (the birth canal) to the upper part of the uterus. The uterus (or the womb) is where a baby grows when a woman is pregnant.

Cervical cancer is preventable with regular screening tests and follow-up. It also is highly curable when found and treated early. Although cervical cancer occurs most often in women over age 30, all women are at risk for cervical cancer. Each year approximately 12,000 women are diagnosed with cervical cancer and 4,000 women die from the disease.[1]

What puts me at greater risk?

The main cause of cervical cancer is the human papillomavirus (HPV), a common virus that can be passed from one person to another during sex. Many people will have an HPV infection at some time in their lives, but because HPV usually goes away on its own, few will get cervical cancer.

Several other factors may affect your risk of developing cervical cancer, including:

- Smoking
- Having HIV, the virus that causes AIDS, or another condition that makes it hard for your body to fight off health problems
- Using birth control pills for a long time
- Having given birth to three or more children

What are the symptoms?

Early on, cervical cancer may not cause signs and symptoms. Advanced cervical cancer may cause bleeding or discharge from the vagina that is not normal for you, such as bleeding after sex. If you have any of these signs, see your doctor, nurse, or health care professional. The symptoms may be caused by something else, but the only way to know is to get checked.

Cervical Cancer Facts

How can I find out if I have cervical cancer?

There are two tests that can help prevent cervical cancer or find it early:

- The **Pap test** (or Pap smear) is one of the most reliable and effective cancer screening tests available. The Pap test only screens for cervical cancer; it does not screen for any other gynecological cancer. It looks for precancers, or cell changes, on the cervix that can be treated, so that cervical cancer is prevented. A Pap test can also identify cervical cancer early, when treatment is most effective. The Pap test is recommended for all women starting at age 21.

- The **HPV test** looks for HPV—the virus that can cause precancerous cell changes and cervical cancer. The HPV test may be used with women aged 30 years and older, or at any age for those who have abnormal Pap test results. Talk with your doctor about whether the HPV test is right for you.

Cervical cancer is preventable with regular screenings, and it is highly treatable if cancer is detected early.

If you are 30 or older, and your screening tests are normal, your chance of getting cervical cancer in the next few years is very low. For that reason, your doctor may tell you that you will not need another screening test for up to three years. If your doctor says that you have cervical cancer, ask to be referred to a gynecologic oncologist—a doctor trained to treat cancers like this. This doctor will work with you to create a treatment plan.

How can I prevent cervical cancer?

There are many ways to prevent or reduce your risk for cervical cancer:

- Get the HPV vaccine. It protects against the types of HPV that most often cause cervical, vaginal, and vulvar cancers, and is recommended for girls and women aged 11 through 26
- See your doctor regularly for a Pap test to find cervical precancerous cells
- Follow up with your doctor if your Pap test results are not normal
- Don't smoke
- Use condoms during sex**
- Limit your number of sexual partners

About the National Breast and Cervical Cancer Early Detection Program (NBCCEDP)

NBCCEDP provides public education, free and low-cost breast and cervical cancer screenings, and diagnostic services to low-income, uninsured, and underserved women. If you have a low income or do not have insurance, you may be able to get a free or low-cost Pap test through the NBCCEDP in your community.

** HPV infection can occur in both male and female genital areas that are covered or protected by a latex condom, as well as in areas that are not covered. While the effect of condoms in preventing HPV infection is unknown, condom use has been associated with a lower rate of cervical cancer.

References

1 U.S. Cancer Statistics Working Group United States Cancer Statistics: 1999 2006 Incidence and Mortality Web based Report. Atlanta, GA: Department of Health and Human Services, Centers for Disease Control and Prevention, and National Cancer Institute; 2010. Available at: http://www.cdc.gov/uscs.

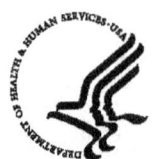 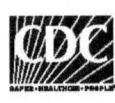

Centers for Disease Control and Prevention
National Breast and Cervical Cancer
Early Detection Program
1 (800) CDC INFO • CDCINFO@cdc.gov
www.cdc.gov/cancer/nbccedp/

CDC's *Inside Knowledge: Get the Facts About Gynecological Cancer* Campaign
www.cdc.gov/cancer/knowledge/

Cervical Cancer Facts

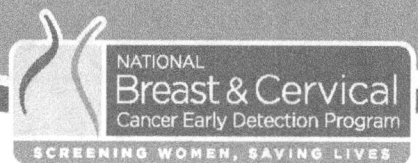

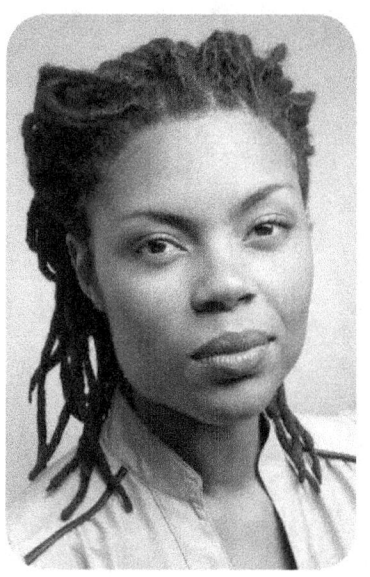

Cervical cancer is the easiest gynecological cancer to prevent with regular screening tests and follow-up. Learn basic information about cervical cancer and how to prevent and recognize it.

What is cervical cancer?

Cancer is a disease in which cells in the body grow out of control. Cancer is always named for the part of the body where it starts, even if it spreads to other body parts later. When cancer starts in the cervix, it is called cervical cancer. The cervix is the lower, narrow end of the uterus. The cervix connects the vagina (the birth canal) to the upper part of the uterus. The uterus (or the womb) is where a baby grows when a woman is pregnant.

Cervical cancer is preventable with regular screening tests and follow-up. It also is highly curable when found and treated early. Although cervical cancer occurs most often in women over age 30, all women are at risk for cervical cancer. Each year approximately 12,000 women are diagnosed with cervical cancer and 4,000 women die from the disease.[1]

What puts me at greater risk?

The main cause of cervical cancer is the human papillomavirus (HPV), a common virus that can be passed from one person to another during sex. Many people will have an HPV infection at some time in their lives, but because HPV usually goes away on its own, few will get cervical cancer.

Several other factors may affect your risk of developing cervical cancer, including:

- Smoking
- Having HIV, the virus that causes AIDS, or another condition that makes it hard for your body to fight off health problems
- Using birth control pills for a long time
- Having given birth to three or more children

What are the symptoms?

Early on, cervical cancer may not cause signs and symptoms. Advanced cervical cancer may cause bleeding or discharge from the vagina that is not normal for you, such as bleeding after sex. If you have any of these signs, see your doctor, nurse, or health care professional. The symptoms may be caused by something else, but the only way to know is to get checked.

Cervical Cancer Facts

How can I find out if I have cervical cancer?

There are two tests that can help prevent cervical cancer or find it early:

- The **Pap test** (or Pap smear) is one of the most reliable and effective cancer screening tests available. The Pap test only screens for cervical cancer; it does not screen for any other gynecological cancer. It looks for precancers, or cell changes, on the cervix that can be treated, so that cervical cancer is prevented. A Pap test can also identify cervical cancer early, when treatment is most effective. The Pap test is recommended for all women starting at age 21.

- The **HPV test** looks for HPV—the virus that can cause precancerous cell changes and cervical cancer. The HPV test may be used with women aged 30 years and older, or at any age for those who have abnormal Pap test results. Talk with your doctor about whether the HPV test is right for you.

Cervical cancer is preventable with regular screenings, and it is highly treatable if cancer is detected early.

If you are 30 or older, and your screening tests are normal, your chance of getting cervical cancer in the next few years is very low. For that reason, your doctor may tell you that you will not need another screening test for up to three years. If your doctor says that you have cervical cancer, ask to be referred to a gynecologic oncologist—a doctor trained to treat cancers like this. This doctor will work with you to create a treatment plan.

How can I prevent cervical cancer?

There are many ways to prevent or reduce your risk for cervical cancer:

- Get the HPV vaccine. It protects against the types of HPV that most often cause cervical, vaginal, and vulvar cancers, and is recommended for girls and women aged 11 through 26
- See your doctor regularly for a Pap test to find cervical precancerous cells
- Follow up with your doctor if your Pap test results are not normal
- Don't smoke
- Use condoms during sex**
- Limit your number of sexual partners

About the National Breast and Cervical Cancer Early Detection Program (NBCCEDP)

NBCCEDP provides public education, free and low-cost breast and cervical cancer screenings, and diagnostic services to low-income, uninsured, and underserved women. If you have a low income or do not have insurance, you may be able to get a free or low-cost Pap test through the NBCCEDP in your community.

** HPV infection can occur in both male and female genital areas that are covered or protected by a latex condom, as well as in areas that are not covered. While the effect of condoms in preventing HPV infection is unknown, condom use has been associated with a lower rate of cervical cancer.

References

1 U.S. Cancer Statistics Working Group. United States Cancer Statistics: 1999_2006 Incidence and Mortality Web_based Report. Atlanta, GA: Department of Health and Human Services, Centers for Disease Control and Prevention, and National Cancer Institute; 2010. Available at: http://www.cdc.gov/uscs.

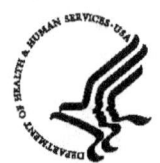
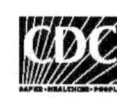

Centers for Disease Control and Prevention
National Breast and Cervical Cancer
Early Detection Program
1 (800) CDC INFO • CDCINFO@cdc.gov
www.cdc.gov/cancer/nbccedp/

CDC's *Inside Knowledge: Get the Facts About Gynecological Cancer* Campaign
www.cdc.gov/cancer/knowledge/

Cervical Cancer Facts

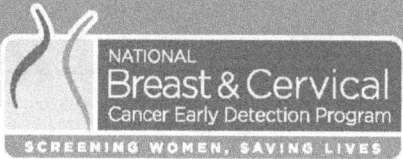

NATIONAL
Breast & Cervical
Cancer Early Detection Program
SCREENING WOMEN, SAVING LIVES

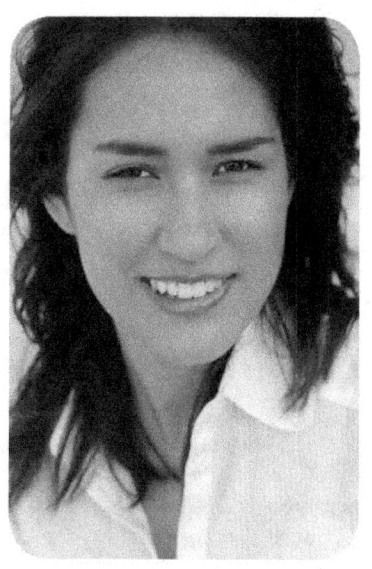

Cervical cancer is the easiest gynecological cancer to prevent with regular screening tests and follow-up. Learn basic information about cervical cancer and how to prevent and recognize it.

What is cervical cancer?

Cancer is a disease in which cells in the body grow out of control. Cancer is always named for the part of the body where it starts, even if it spreads to other body parts later. When cancer starts in the cervix, it is called cervical cancer. The cervix is the lower, narrow end of the uterus. The cervix connects the vagina (the birth canal) to the upper part of the uterus. The uterus (or the womb) is where a baby grows when a woman is pregnant.

Cervical cancer is preventable with regular screening tests and follow-up. It also is highly curable when found and treated early. Although cervical cancer occurs most often in women over age 30, all women are at risk for cervical cancer. Each year approximately 12,000 women are diagnosed with cervical cancer and 4,000 women die from the disease.[1]

What puts me at greater risk?

The main cause of cervical cancer is the human papillomavirus (HPV), a common virus that can be passed from one person to another during sex. Many people will have an HPV infection at some time in their lives, but because HPV usually goes away on its own, few will get cervical cancer.

Several other factors may affect your risk of developing cervical cancer, including:

- Smoking
- Having HIV, the virus that causes AIDS, or another condition that makes it hard for your body to fight off health problems
- Using birth control pills for a long time
- Having given birth to three or more children

What are the symptoms?

Early on, cervical cancer may not cause signs and symptoms. Advanced cervical cancer may cause bleeding or discharge from the vagina that is not normal for you, such as bleeding after sex. If you have any of these signs, see your doctor, nurse, or health care professional. The symptoms may be caused by something else, but the only way to know is to get checked.

Cervical Cancer Facts

How can I find out if I have cervical cancer?

There are two tests that can help prevent cervical cancer or find it early:

- The **Pap test** (or Pap smear) is one of the most reliable and effective cancer screening tests available. The Pap test only screens for cervical cancer; it does not screen for any other gynecological cancer. It looks for precancers, or cell changes, on the cervix that can be treated, so that cervical cancer is prevented. A Pap test can also identify cervical cancer early, when treatment is most effective. The Pap test is recommended for all women starting at age 21.

- The **HPV test** looks for HPV—the virus that can cause precancerous cell changes and cervical cancer. The HPV test may be used with women aged 30 years and older, or at any age for those who have abnormal Pap test results. Talk with your doctor about whether the HPV test is right for you.

Cervical cancer is preventable with regular screenings, and it is highly treatable if cancer is detected early.

If you are 30 or older, and your screening tests are normal, your chance of getting cervical cancer in the next few years is very low. For that reason, your doctor may tell you that you will not need another screening test for up to three years. If your doctor says that you have cervical cancer, ask to be referred to a gynecologic oncologist—a doctor trained to treat cancers like this. This doctor will work with you to create a treatment plan.

How can I prevent cervical cancer?

There are many ways to prevent or reduce your risk for cervical cancer:

- Get the HPV vaccine. It protects against the types of HPV that most often cause cervical, vaginal, and vulvar cancers, and is recommended for girls and women aged 11 through 26
- See your doctor regularly for a Pap test to find cervical precancerous cells
- Follow up with your doctor if your Pap test results are not normal
- Don't smoke
- Use condoms during sex**
- Limit your number of sexual partners

About the National Breast and Cervical Cancer Early Detection Program (NBCCEDP)

NBCCEDP provides public education, free and low-cost breast and cervical cancer screenings, and diagnostic services to low-income, uninsured, and underserved women. If you have a low income or do not have insurance, you may be able to get a free or low-cost Pap test through the NBCCEDP in your community.

** HPV infection can occur in both male and female genital areas that are covered or protected by a latex condom, as well as in areas that are not covered. While the effect of condoms in preventing HPV infection is unknown, condom use has been associated with a lower rate of cervical cancer.

References

1 U.S. Cancer Statistics Working Group. United States Cancer Statistics: 1999 2006 Incidence and Mortality Web based Report. Atlanta, GA: Department of Health and Human Services, Centers for Disease Control and Prevention, and National Cancer Institute; 2010. Available at: http://www.cdc.gov/uscs.

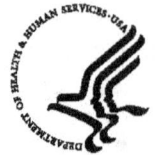
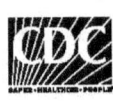

Centers for Disease Control and Prevention
National Breast and Cervical Cancer
Early Detection Program
1 (800) CDC INFO • CDCINFO@cdc.gov
www.cdc.gov/cancer/nbccedp/

CDC's *Inside Knowledge: Get the Facts About Gynecological Cancer* Campaign
www.cdc.gov/cancer/knowledge/

Cervical Cancer Facts

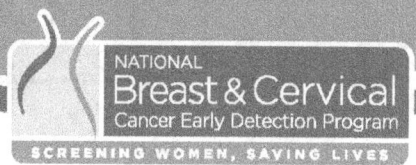

NATIONAL
Breast & Cervical
Cancer Early Detection Program
SCREENING WOMEN, SAVING LIVES

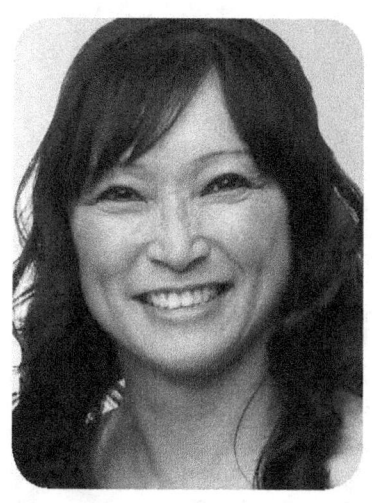

Cervical cancer is the easiest gynecological cancer to prevent with regular screening tests and follow-up. Learn basic information about cervical cancer and how to prevent and recognize it.

What is cervical cancer?

Cancer is a disease in which cells in the body grow out of control. Cancer is always named for the part of the body where it starts, even if it spreads to other body parts later. When cancer starts in the cervix, it is called cervical cancer. The cervix is the lower, narrow end of the uterus. The cervix connects the vagina (the birth canal) to the upper part of the uterus. The uterus (or the womb) is where a baby grows when a woman is pregnant.

Cervical cancer is preventable with regular screening tests and follow-up. It also is highly curable when found and treated early. Although cervical cancer occurs most often in women over age 30, all women are at risk for cervical cancer. Each year approximately 12,000 women are diagnosed with cervical cancer and 4,000 women die from the disease.[1]

What puts me at greater risk?

The main cause of cervical cancer is the human papillomavirus (HPV), a common virus that can be passed from one person to another during sex. Many people will have an HPV infection at some time in their lives, but because HPV usually goes away on its own, few will get cervical cancer.

Several other factors may affect your risk of developing cervical cancer, including:

- Smoking
- Having HIV, the virus that causes AIDS, or another condition that makes it hard for your body to fight off health problems
- Using birth control pills for a long time
- Having given birth to three or more children

What are the symptoms?

Early on, cervical cancer may not cause signs and symptoms. Advanced cervical cancer may cause bleeding or discharge from the vagina that is not normal for you, such as bleeding after sex. If you have any of these signs, see your doctor, nurse, or health care professional. The symptoms may be caused by something else, but the only way to know is to get checked.

Cervical Cancer Facts

How can I find out if I have cervical cancer?

There are two tests that can help prevent cervical cancer or find it early:

- The **Pap test** (or Pap smear) is one of the most reliable and effective cancer screening tests available. The Pap test only screens for cervical cancer; it does not screen for any other gynecological cancer. It looks for precancers, or cell changes, on the cervix that can be treated, so that cervical cancer is prevented. A Pap test can also identify cervical cancer early, when treatment is most effective. The Pap test is recommended for all women starting at age 21.

- The **HPV test** looks for HPV—the virus that can cause precancerous cell changes and cervical cancer. The HPV test may be used with women aged 30 years and older, or at any age for those who have abnormal Pap test results. Talk with your doctor about whether the HPV test is right for you.

Cervical cancer is preventable with regular screenings, and it is highly treatable if cancer is detected early.

If you are 30 or older, and your screening tests are normal, your chance of getting cervical cancer in the next few years is very low. For that reason, your doctor may tell you that you will not need another screening test for up to three years. If your doctor says that you have cervical cancer, ask to be referred to a gynecologic oncologist—a doctor trained to treat cancers like this. This doctor will work with you to create a treatment plan.

How can I prevent cervical cancer?

There are many ways to prevent or reduce your risk for cervical cancer:

- Get the HPV vaccine. It protects against the types of HPV that most often cause cervical, vaginal, and vulvar cancers, and is recommended for girls and women aged 11 through 26
- See your doctor regularly for a Pap test to find cervical precancerous cells
- Follow up with your doctor if your Pap test results are not normal
- Don't smoke
- Use condoms during sex**
- Limit your number of sexual partners

About the National Breast and Cervical Cancer Early Detection Program (NBCCEDP)

NBCCEDP provides public education, free and low-cost breast and cervical cancer screenings, and diagnostic services to low-income, uninsured, and underserved women. If you have a low income or do not have insurance, you may be able to get a free or low-cost Pap test through the NBCCEDP in your community.

** HPV infection can occur in both male and female genital areas that are covered or protected by a latex condom, as well as in areas that are not covered. While the effect of condoms in preventing HPV infection is unknown, condom use has been associated with a lower rate of cervical cancer.

References

1 U.S. Cancer Statistics Working Group. United States Cancer Statistics: 1999 2006 Incidence and Mortality Web based Report. Atlanta, GA: Department of Health and Human Services, Centers for Disease Control and Prevention, and National Cancer Institute; 2010. Available at: http://www.cdc.gov/uscs.

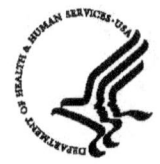
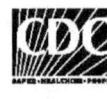

Centers for Disease Control and Prevention
National Breast and Cervical Cancer
Early Detection Program
1 (800) CDC INFO • CDCINFO@cdc.gov
www.cdc.gov/cancer/nbccedp/

CDC's *Inside Knowledge: Get the Facts About Gynecological Cancer* Campaign
www.cdc.gov/cancer/knowledge/

Cervical Cancer Facts

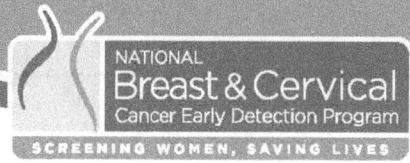

NATIONAL
Breast & Cervical
Cancer Early Detection Program
SCREENING WOMEN, SAVING LIVES

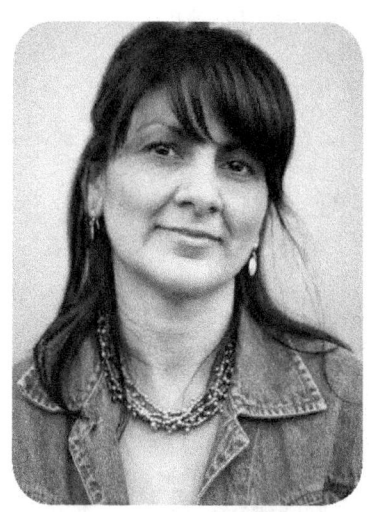

Cervical cancer is the easiest gynecological cancer to prevent with regular screening tests and follow-up. Learn basic information about cervical cancer and how to prevent and recognize it.

What is cervical cancer?

Cancer is a disease in which cells in the body grow out of control. Cancer is always named for the part of the body where it starts, even if it spreads to other body parts later. When cancer starts in the cervix, it is called cervical cancer. The cervix is the lower, narrow end of the uterus. The cervix connects the vagina (the birth canal) to the upper part of the uterus. The uterus (or the womb) is where a baby grows when a woman is pregnant.

Cervical cancer is preventable with regular screening tests and follow-up. It also is highly curable when found and treated early. Although cervical cancer occurs most often in women over age 30, all women are at risk for cervical cancer. Each year approximately 12,000 women are diagnosed with cervical cancer and 4,000 women die from the disease.[1]

What puts me at greater risk?

The main cause of cervical cancer is the human papillomavirus (HPV), a common virus that can be passed from one person to another during sex. Many people will have an HPV infection at some time in their lives, but because HPV usually goes away on its own, few will get cervical cancer.

Several other factors may affect your risk of developing cervical cancer, including:

- Smoking
- Having HIV, the virus that causes AIDS, or another condition that makes it hard for your body to fight off health problems
- Using birth control pills for a long time
- Having given birth to three or more children

What are the symptoms?

Early on, cervical cancer may not cause signs and symptoms. Advanced cervical cancer may cause bleeding or discharge from the vagina that is not normal for you, such as bleeding after sex. If you have any of these signs, see your doctor, nurse, or health care professional. The symptoms may be caused by something else, but the only way to know is to get checked.

Cervical Cancer Facts

How can I find out if I have cervical cancer?

There are two tests that can help prevent cervical cancer or find it early:

- The **Pap test** (or Pap smear) is one of the most reliable and effective cancer screening tests available. The Pap test only screens for cervical cancer; it does not screen for any other gynecological cancer. It looks for precancers, or cell changes, on the cervix that can be treated, so that cervical cancer is prevented. A Pap test can also identify cervical cancer early, when treatment is most effective. The Pap test is recommended for all women starting at age 21.

- The **HPV test** looks for HPV—the virus that can cause precancerous cell changes and cervical cancer. The HPV test may be used with women aged 30 years and older, or at any age for those who have abnormal Pap test results. Talk with your doctor about whether the HPV test is right for you.

Cervical cancer is preventable with regular screenings, and it is highly treatable if cancer is detected early.

If you are 30 or older, and your screening tests are normal, your chance of getting cervical cancer in the next few years is very low. For that reason, your doctor may tell you that you will not need another screening test for up to three years. If your doctor says that you have cervical cancer, ask to be referred to a gynecologic oncologist—a doctor trained to treat cancers like this. This doctor will work with you to create a treatment plan.

How can I prevent cervical cancer?

There are many ways to prevent or reduce your risk for cervical cancer:

- Get the HPV vaccine. It protects against the types of HPV that most often cause cervical, vaginal, and vulvar cancers, and is recommended for girls and women aged 11 through 26
- See your doctor regularly for a Pap test to find cervical precancerous cells
- Follow up with your doctor if your Pap test results are not normal
- Don't smoke
- Use condoms during sex**
- Limit your number of sexual partners

About the National Breast and Cervical Cancer Early Detection Program (NBCCEDP)

NBCCEDP provides public education, free and low-cost breast and cervical cancer screenings, and diagnostic services to low-income, uninsured, and underserved women. If you have a low income or do not have insurance, you may be able to get a free or low-cost Pap test through the NBCCEDP in your community.

** HPV infection can occur in both male and female genital areas that are covered or protected by a latex condom, as well as in areas that are not covered. While the effect of condoms in preventing HPV infection is unknown, condom use has been associated with a lower rate of cervical cancer.

References

1 U.S. Cancer Statistics Working Group. United States Cancer Statistics: 1999–2006 Incidence and Mortality Web-based Report. Atlanta, GA: Department of Health and Human Services, Centers for Disease Control and Prevention, and National Cancer Institute; 2010. Available at: http://www.cdc.gov/uscs.

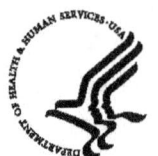 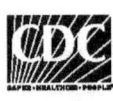

Centers for Disease Control and Prevention
National Breast and Cervical Cancer
Early Detection Program
1 (800) CDC INFO • CDCINFO@cdc.gov
www.cdc.gov/cancer/nbccedp/

CDC's *Inside Knowledge: Get the Facts About Gynecological Cancer* Campaign
www.cdc.gov/cancer/knowledge/

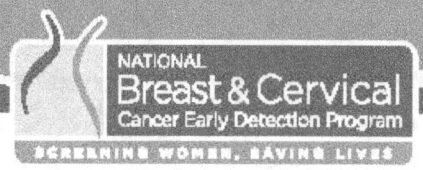

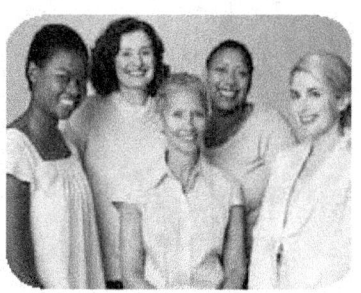

Why You Should Partner with NBCCEDP Programs

The Centers for Disease Control and Prevention's National Breast and Cervical Cancer Early Detection Program (NBCCEDP) provides consumer education, free and low-cost breast and cervical cancer screenings, and diagnostic services to low-income, uninsured, and underserved women. For the past 20 years, NBCCEDP has served more than 3.7 million women and provided more than 9.2 million screening examinations through grants provided to programs in all 50 states, the District of Columbia, five U.S. territories, and 12 American Indian and Alaskan Native tribal organizations.[1]

Why does our program need partners?

Federal funding alone cannot fully sustain the life-saving services we offer at the program services level—partner support is needed. As an NBCCEDP program, we are required to match every $3 of federal funds we receive with $1 of non-federal resources (monetary or in-kind). In addition, more women are in need of NBCCEDP services than in years past, meaning our program needs resources now, more than ever before.

How can you benefit from a partnership with us?

Your support can help our program provide consumer education, as well as free and low-cost breast and cervical cancer-related services to women in need. In addition to helping keep women healthy, your organization also benefits from:

- Positively impacting corporate reputation by raising visibility as a caring member of the community. Breast and cervical cancer affect everyone, so a connection to this cause will be meaningful to your employees and constituents.

- Knowing your support will directly benefit women in your state or community. This is a clear indication of corporate citizenship.

- Linking to a credible and highly respected breast and cervical cancer program.

- Increasing valuable marketing, promotion, public relations, and networking opportunities. By collaborating with our program, your organization can show its goodwill through connecting your brand with a good cause, word-of-mouth exposure to new audiences, materials sharing, and press coverage of local events.

- Differentiation from competitors who have not demonstrated corporate responsibility.

Collectively, these benefits also can help your organization achieve its goals and objectives, such as driving sales or attracting members.

If your organization is already involved with women's issues or cancer, take this opportunity to leverage current efforts and investments by further connecting to the cause to increase chances for impact and return on investment.

What can partners do to help?

Partners—including local businesses, corporations, health care providers, faith-based organizations, community-based organizations, and many others— can provide a range of in-kind and monetary support to help women access critically needed breast and cervical cancer-related services. Examples of partner contributions include consumer education, provider education, direct funding, printing, translation, recruitment, fundraising, meeting facility provision, and advocacy.

Our program has a range of unique needs and can benefit from strong partnerships of any size or scale. No contribution is too small.

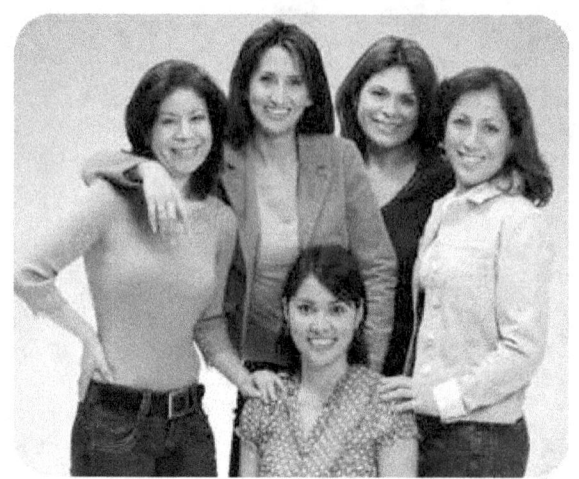

References

1 Centers for Disease Control and Prevention, National Breast and Cervical Cancer Early Detection Program. *Minimum Data Elements*. April 2010.

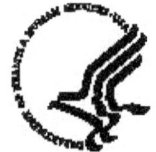 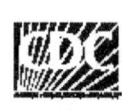

Centers for Disease Control and Prevention
National Breast and Cervical Cancer
Early Detection Program
1 (800) CDC INFO • CDCINFO@cdc.gov
www.cdc.gov/cancer/nbccedp/

Why You Should Partner with NBCCEDP Programs

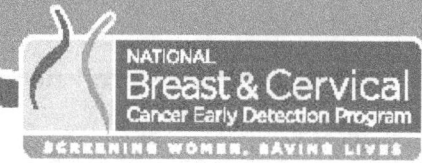

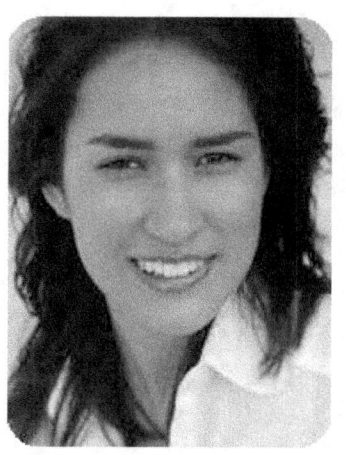

Why You Should Partner with NBCCEDP Programs

The Centers for Disease Control and Prevention's National Breast and Cervical Cancer Early Detection Program (NBCCEDP) provides consumer education, free and low-cost breast and cervical cancer screenings, and diagnostic services to low-income, uninsured, and underserved women. For the past 20 years, NBCCEDP has served more than 3.7 million women and provided more than 9.2 million screening examinations through grants provided to programs in all 50 states, the District of Columbia, five U.S. territories, and 12 American Indian and Alaskan Native tribal organizations.[1]

Why does our program need partners?

Federal funding alone cannot fully sustain the life-saving services we offer at the program services level—partner support is needed. As an NBCCEDP program, we are required to match every $3 of federal funds we receive with $1 of non-federal resources (monetary or in-kind). In addition, more women are in need of NBCCEDP services than in years past, meaning our program needs resources now, more than ever before.

How can you benefit from a partnership with us?

Your support can help our program provide consumer education, as well as free and low-cost breast and cervical cancer-related services to women in need. In addition to helping keep women healthy, your organization also benefits from:

- Positively impacting corporate reputation by raising visibility as a caring member of the community. Breast and cervical cancer affect everyone, so a connection to this cause will be meaningful to your employees and constituents.

- Knowing your support will directly benefit women in your state or community. This is a clear indication of corporate citizenship.

- Linking to a credible and highly respected breast and cervical cancer program.

- Increasing valuable marketing, promotion, public relations, and networking opportunities. By collaborating with our program, your organization can show its goodwill through connecting your brand with a good cause, word-of-mouth exposure to new audiences, materials sharing, and press coverage of local events.

- Differentiation from competitors who have not demonstrated corporate responsibility.

Collectively, these benefits also can help your organization achieve its goals and objectives, such as driving sales or attracting members.

If your organization is already involved with women's issues or cancer, take this opportunity to leverage current efforts and investments by further connecting to the cause to increase chances for impact and return on investment.

What can partners do to help?

Partners—including local businesses, corporations, health care providers, faith-based organizations, community-based organizations, and many others—can provide a range of in-kind and monetary support to help women access critically needed breast and cervical cancer-related services. Examples of partner contributions include consumer education, provider education, direct funding, printing, translation, recruitment, fundraising, meeting facility provision, and advocacy.

Our program has a range of unique needs and can benefit from strong partnerships of any size or scale. No contribution is too small.

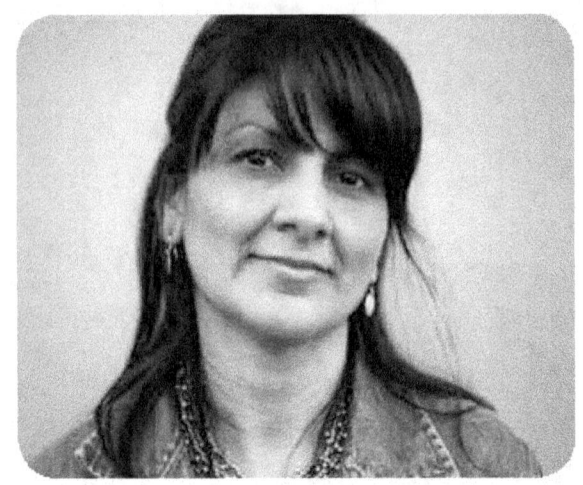

References

1 Centers for Disease Control and Prevention, National Breast and Cervical Cancer Early Detection Program. *Minimum Data Elements*. April 2010.

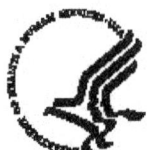 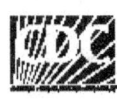

Centers for Disease Control and Prevention
National Breast and Cervical Cancer
Early Detection Program
1 (800) CDC INFO • CDCINFO@cdc.gov
www.cdc.gov/cancer/nbccedp/

Your Program Name

Program overview information to be inserted in this space.

Program at a Glance
Month/Day/Year to Month/Day/Year

Total Number of Women Served	TBD
Number of Eligible Women in Service Area	TBD
Percent of Eligible Women Served	TBD

Program Eligibility Requirements

Age (Breast Screening)	TBD
Age (Cervical Screening)	TBD
Income	TBD
Insurance	TBD

Age Range of Women Served*

Age	Breast %	Cervical %
18 to 39 years	TBD	TBD
40 to 49 years	TBD	TBD
50 to 64 years	TBD	TBD
>64 years	TBD	TBD

Race/Ethnicity of Women Served vs. Population Segment

Race/Ethnicity	Program %	Population %
White	TBD	TBD
Black	TBD	TBD
Hispanic	TBD	TBD
Asian/Pacific Islander	TBD	TBD
American Indian	TBD	TBD
Other Unknown	TBD	TBD
>1 Race	TBD	TBD

About the National Breast and Cervical Cancer Early Detection Program

The Centers for Disease Control and Prevention's National Breast and Cervical Cancer Early Detection Program (NBCCEDP) provides consumer education, free and low-cost breast and cervical cancer screenings, and diagnostic services to low-income, uninsured, and underserved women. The NBCCEDP provides funding to all 50 states, the District of Columbia, 5 U.S. territories, and 12 American Indian/Alaska Native tribes or tribal organizations. Since 1991, NBCCEDP grantee programs have served more than 3.7 million women, and provided more than 9.2 million breast and cervical cancer screening examinations.

Federal guidelines establish eligibility to uninsured and underinsured women at or below 250% of federal poverty level, ages 18–64 for cervical cancer screening and 40–64 for breast cancer screening.

Month/Year

Screening History of Women Served

Screening History	Program %**
Never Had a Mammogram	TBD
Never Had a Pap Test	TBD

Number of Screening Procedures Performed: TBD

Clinical Breast Exams	TBD
Screening Mammograms	TBD
Pap Test	TBD

Total Diagnoses: TBD

Breast Cancer	
Non-invasive Cancer	TBD
Invasive Cancer	TBD
Cervical Dysplasia and Invasive Cervical Cancer	
Mild Dysplasia/CIN 1	TBD
Moderate Dysplasia/CIN 2, 3	TBD
Severe Dysplasia/CIS, AIS	TBD
Invasive Cancer	TBD

*Columns total 100%

** This percentage represents the number of women who had never been screened at the time of enrollment.

Program Contact Information Here.

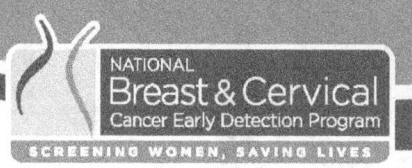

Thank You Letter and Recognition Certificate

It is important to recognize partner support and share results of their contributions. Partners may feel buoyed learning the impact of their support to your program. The following sample Thank You Letter and Recognition Certificate can be shared with current and new partners to demonstrate the impact of their support and reinforce how meaningful it is to your program.

SAMPLE THANK YOU LETTER

Dear **[PARTNER CONTACT'S NAME]**,

On behalf of **[PROGRAM NAME]**, I would like to thank you for **[PARTNER ORGANIZATION NAME]** **[CONTRIBUTION]**. Because of your partnership, we **[PROVIDE SPECIFIC RESULTS IF AVAILABLE (e.g., reached X more women with education materials, screened X more women, trained X community outreach workers)]**.

Each year, more than 200,000 women are diagnosed with breast and cervical cancer combined. As part of the Centers for Disease Control and Prevention's National Breast and Cervical Cancer Early Detection Program, we provide women in need with education, and free and low-cost breast and cervical cancer screenings and diagnostic services. Support from organizations like **[PARTNER ORGANIZATION NAME]** helps us continue our mission with **[STATE]** women. Together, our work helps save lives through early detection of breast and cervical cancer.

We look forward to working together on future efforts.

Thank you,

[SIGNATURE]
[NAME]
[TITLE]
[PROGRAM NAME]

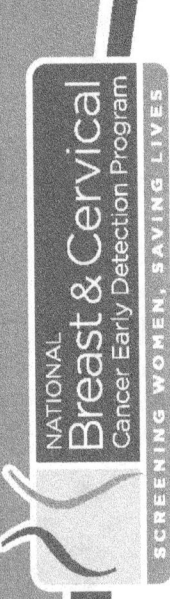

NATIONAL
Breast & Cervical
Cancer Early Detection Program
SCREENING WOMEN, SAVING LIVES

Certificate of Recognition

PRESENTED TO

[PARTNER NAME]

In honor of your contributions to

[PROGRAM NAME]

to help save lives through early detection of breast and cervical cancer.

[MONTH DAY, YEAR]

[Name, Title,
Organization]

Technical Instructions for Customizing Materials

These instructions apply to the "Materials for Distribution by Programs" within this toolkit. All of these materials can be customized with your program's information and logo. The *Certificate for Recognition* and *Program Profile Template* have additional customizable fields.

Note: Adobe Acrobat Reader is required for adding text-only program information and data. Your program or a vendor (e.g., a quick-print or design shop) will need to have Adobe Acrobat Standard or Professional to add a logo to these materials.

HOW TO INSERT TEXT-ONLY INFORMATION: Click on the field you would like to customize. Type your program's information into the customizable text boxes throughout these materials.

HOW TO INSERT YOUR PROGRAM LOGO: NOTE: Logo files should be vector EPS files, or JPEG or TIFF files that are a minimum of 300 dpi.

1) Since the materials are saved for Adobe Acrobat Reader users, you will first need to activate the editable logo fields in Adobe Acrobat Standard or Professional. To do this, click on "Forms" from the tool bar menu at the top of the page once you've opened the document you'd like to add your logo to. Select "Add or Edit Fields..." A message box will appear, please click "Save a Copy." Save a copy of the file in a preferred folder.

2) Close the Adobe Acrobat file that is currently open and open the version of the document from the folder where you saved it. Click on "Forms" from the tool bar again, and select "Add or Edit Fields." You will now see that all the fields are active.

3) Double click on the "Program Logo" box in the document. A "Button Properties" box will appear. Click on the "Options" tab. Then, click the "Choose Icon" button in the lower right corner.

4) Click on the "Browse" button in the top right of the select icon box and then locate the logo file on your computer. NOTE: Once you select "Browse" you will need to select your logo's file type from the drop down menu at the bottom of the page (either Postcript/EPS, JPEG, or TIFF) when searching for the logo file.

5) Select your logo file and click the "Select" button. Your logo will appear in the customizable box. Click "OK" and then, in the next window, click "Close." Your program logo will now be embedded into the document. For the *Program Profile Template* only, repeat steps 3 through 5 to add a logo to the second page.

IMPORTANT: Do not attempt to move or edit any other fields while in "Add or Edit Fields" mode. Once you have added your logo, click on "Forms" in the tool bar again, and select "Close Form Editing."

7) Your file is now ready to print.

FACT SHEETS

PAGE 1

PAGE 2

In this space, consider adding your program's logo. Refer to detailed instructions for adding logos above.

Include your program name and contact information (e.g., phone number, website, and/or mailing address).

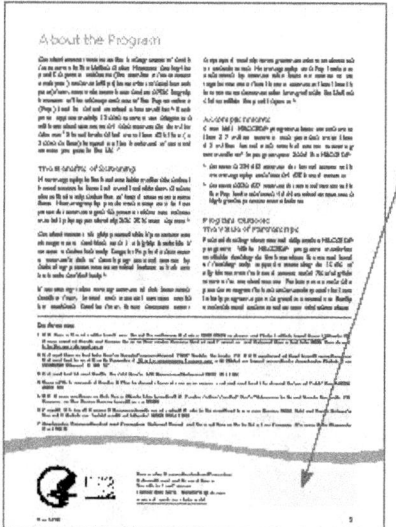

CERTIFICATE OF RECOGNITION

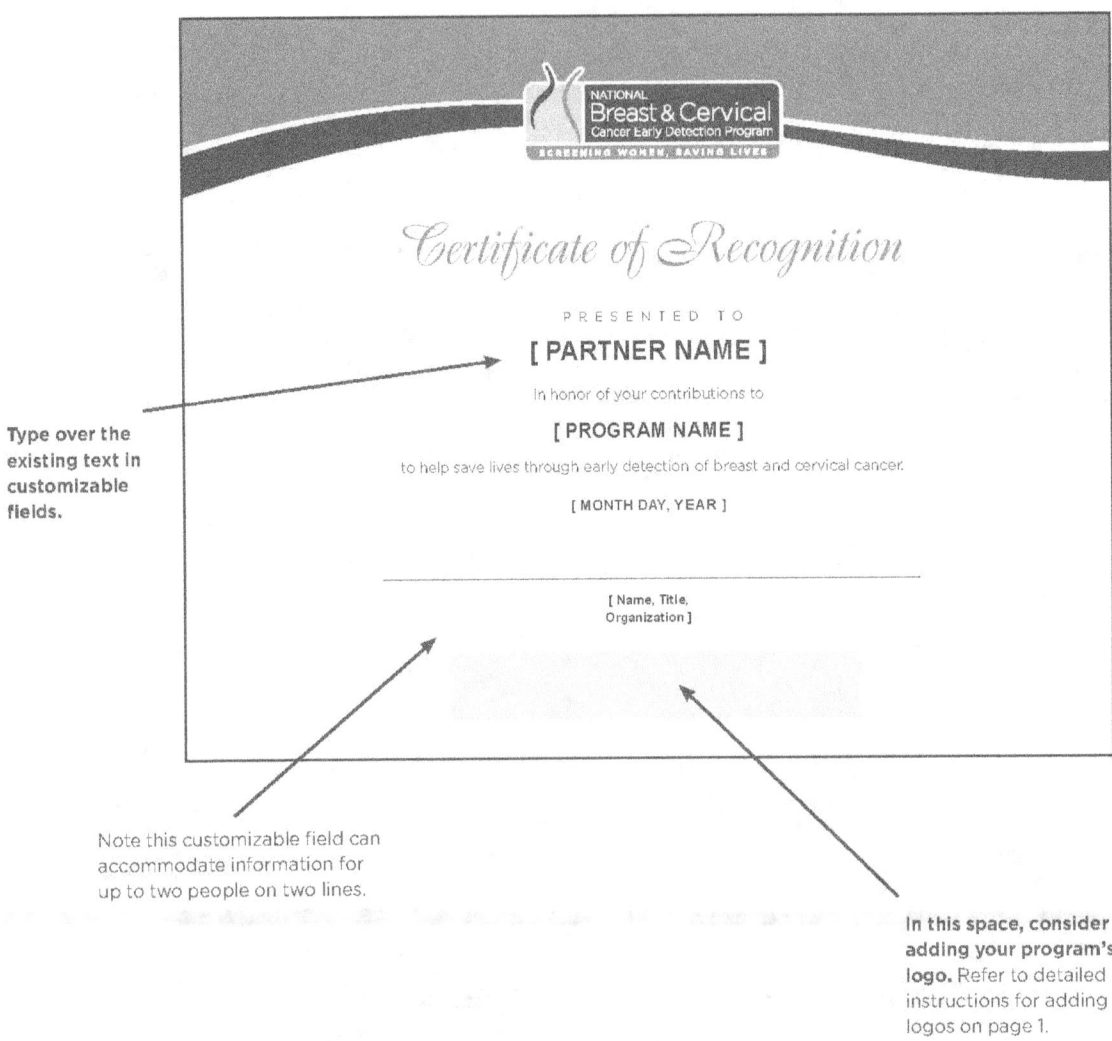

Type over the existing text in customizable fields.

Note this customizable field can accommodate information for up to two people on two lines.

In this space, consider adding your program's logo. Refer to detailed instructions for adding logos on page 1.

Engaging, Building, Expanding: An NBCCEDP Partnership Development Toolkit
Materials for Distribution by Programs: Technical Instructions for Customizing Materials

March 2011

2

PROGRAM PROFILE TEMPLATE

PAGE 1

Insert your program name here.

Include a 150 word overview of your program in the space provided. Consider including information such as what year your program began receiving funding through NBCCEDP, the total number of women screened since the program's inception, priority audiences, details about your program's specific eligibility requirements, number of women served with partner funds/ support, or other information.

In this space, consider adding your program's logo. Refer to detailed instructions for adding logos on page 1.

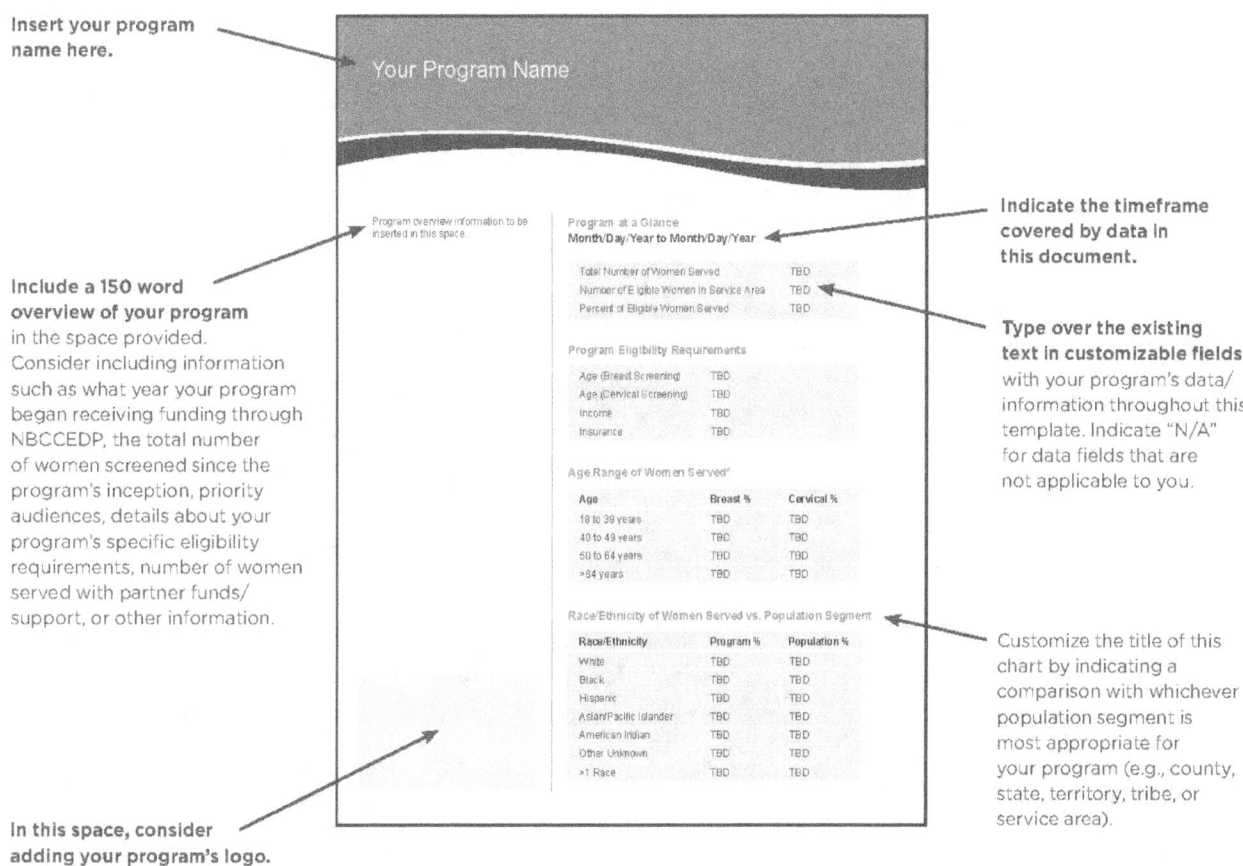

Indicate the timeframe covered by data in this document.

Type over the existing text in customizable fields with your program's data/ information throughout this template. Indicate "N/A" for data fields that are not applicable to you.

Customize the title of this chart by indicating a comparison with whichever population segment is most appropriate for your program (e.g., county, state, territory, tribe, or service area).

Engaging, Building, Expanding: An NBCCEDP Partnership Development Toolkit
Materials for Distribution by Programs: Technical Instructions for Customizing Materials

March 2011

3

PROGRAM PROFILE TEMPLATE

PAGE 2

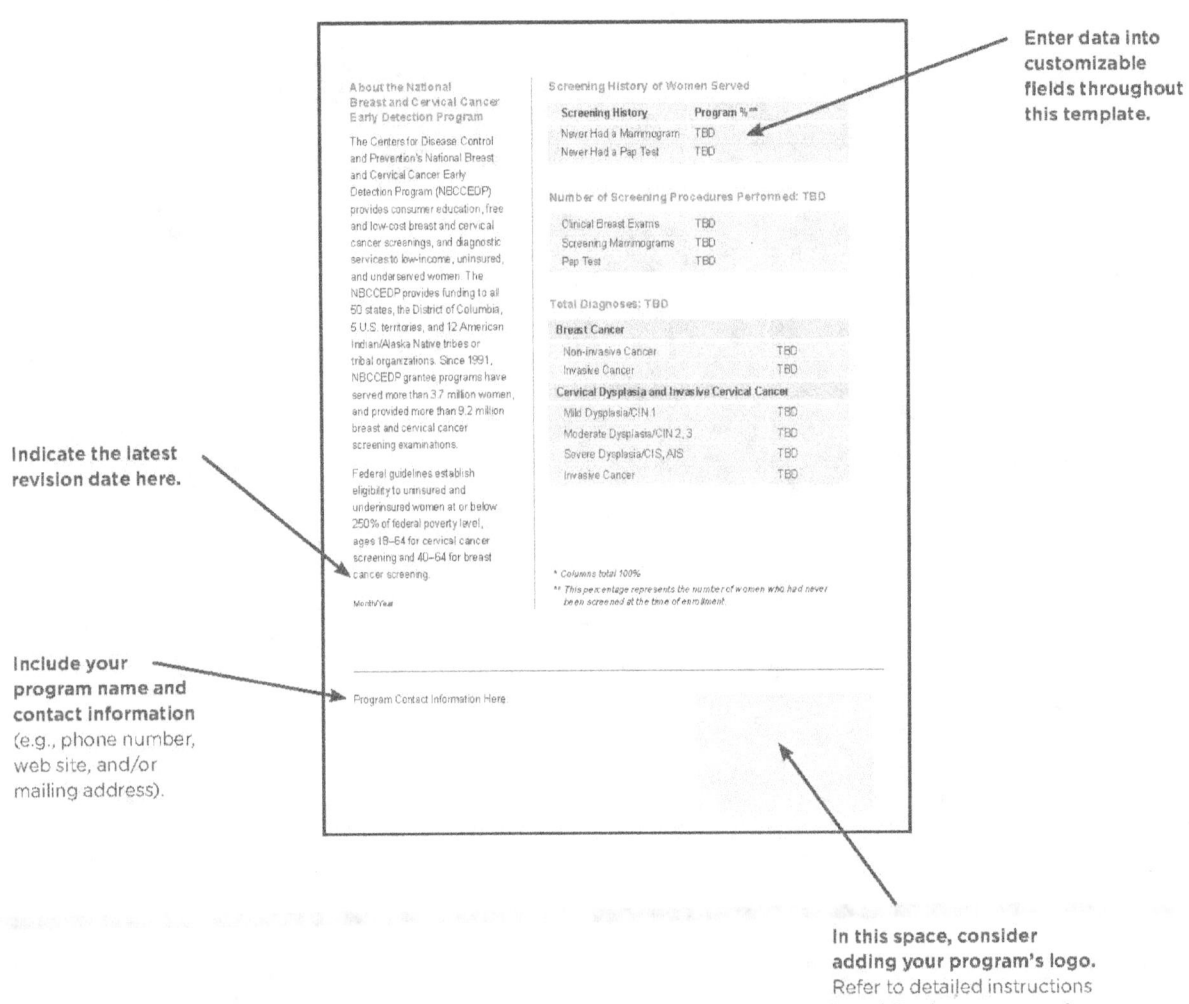

Enter data into customizable fields throughout this template.

Indicate the latest revision date here.

Include your program name and contact information (e.g., phone number, web site, and/or mailing address).

In this space, consider adding your program's logo. Refer to detailed instructions for adding logos on page 1.

Engaging, Building, Expanding: An NBCCEDP Partnership Development Toolkit
Materials for Distribution by Programs: Technical Instructions for Customizing Materials

March 2011

4

National Breast and Cervical Cancer Early Detection Program
Brand Identity Usage Terms and Conditions

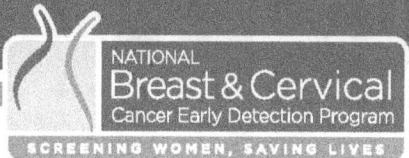

The National Breast and Cervical Cancer Early Detection Program (NBCCEDP) provides public education, free and low-cost breast and cervical cancer screenings, and diagnostic services to low-income, uninsured, and underserved women.

This expanded guide was created to protect the NBCCEDP brand and ensure that program partners employ the national NBCCEDP Brand Identity, 20th Anniversary Brand Identity, text badge, typefaces, and color palette in a consistent manner.

> In order to use the NBCCEDP brand identities on materials, a Brand Identity Agreement Form must be submitted to the CDC in advance. Use of the text badge does not require you to submit this form.
>
> Using the NBCCEDP brand identities or text badge to affiliate with the national program is not a requirement, however, all uses must comply with these Usage Terms and Conditions outlined below and on the following pages.

NBCCEDP Brand Identities and Program Name

The following pages show the approved brand identity standards and graphic requirements for two brand identity treatments (NBCCEDP Brand Identity and 20th Anniversary Brand Identity) and instructions on affiliating with the national program.

Important:

— Building awareness and recognition of NBCCEDP means the name and brand identity must stay the same every time they are seen or heard.

— Never change the NBCCEDP name by adding or appending additional words or meaning.

— When spelled out, the term National Breast and Cervical Cancer Early Detection Program must appear with initial caps. The acronym NBCCEDP must appear in all caps at all times.

NBCCEDP Colors

There are two colors that are represented in most NBCCEDP communications to exemplify the NBCCEDP brand, in addition to silver and black.

— **Teal:** Represents cervical cancer

— **Pink:** Represents breast cancer

When associating with the national program, you must use only the official brand identities provided with these colors, or the black and white versions.

National Breast and Cervical Cancer Early Detection Program
NBCCEDP Brand Identity Standards

This guide was created to protect the NBCCEDP brand and ensure that program partners employ the national brand identity, typefaces, and color palette in a consistent manner.

NBCCEDP BRAND IDENTITY ELEMENTS

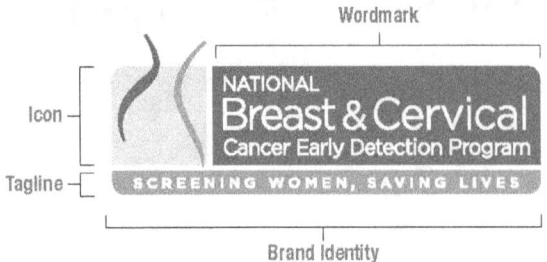

Wordmark

Icon

Tagline

Brand Identity

Any use of the Wordmark and Tagline as separate items requires prior approval.

Brand Identity Fonts
Wordmark font: Gotham Light
Tagline font: Gotham Bold

NBCCEDP COLOR USES

To maintain the integrity of the NBCCEDP Brand Identity and ensure consistency in all usage, the colors specified below must be used when printing in four-color process. As readability is of utmost importance, it is critical to use the proper colors for a dark or light background, as shown.

CMYK-Color Brand Identity

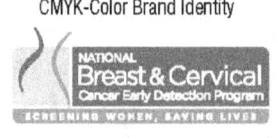
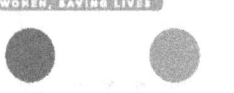
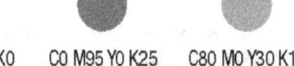

C0 M22 Y0 K0   C0 M95 Y0 K25   C80 M0 Y30 K10

1-Color Brand Identity (black)

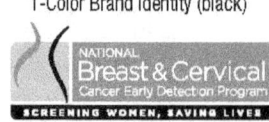
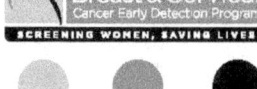

30%   60%   100%

NBCCEDP BACKGROUND COLOR USE

Use the CMYK-color or 1-color (black) version of the NBCCEDP Brand Identity when applying it to a white or light/mid-tone background. (See examples below)

Use the CMYK-color or 1-color (black) version with white rule outline of the NBCCEDP Brand Identity when applying it to a mid/dark-tone or dark background. (See examples below)

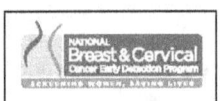
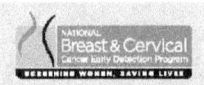
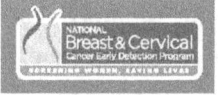
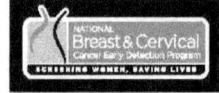

White Background   Light/Mid-tone Background   Mid/Dark-tone Background   Dark Background

SIZING AND POSITIONING

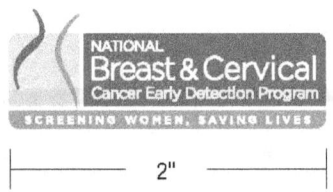

2"

Brand identity should never be smaller than 2" wide.

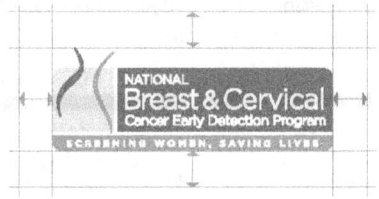

Leave clear space approximately 1/4" on all sides of the brand identity.

PROHIBITED USES

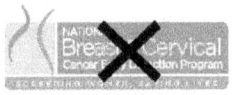
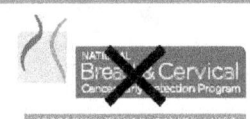
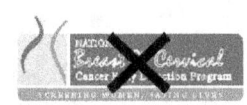
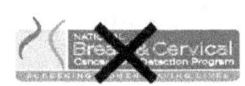

Do not alter the color of the brand identity.

Do not alter the position of the brand identity.

Do not alter or substitute the Wordmark or Tagline font from its existing form.

Brand identity must be re-sized in correct proportion.

March 2011

National Breast and Cervical Cancer Early Detection Program
NBCCEDP 20th Anniversary Brand Identity Standards

NBCCEDP developed the 20th Anniversary Brand Identity to celebrate 20 years of success. This guide was created to ensure that NBCCEDP partners employ this brand identity, typefaces, and color palette in a consistent manner.

NBCCEDP BRAND IDENTITY ELEMENTS

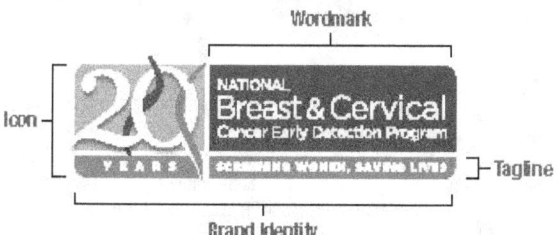

Wordmark · Icon · Tagline · Brand Identity

Any use of the Wordmark and Tagline as separate items requires prior approval.

Brand Identity Fonts
Wordmark font: Gotham Light
Tagline font: Gotham Bold

NBCCEDP COLOR USES

To maintain the integrity of the NBCCEDP 20th Anniversary Brand Identity and ensure consistency in all usage, the colors specified below must be used when printing in four-color process. As readability is of utmost importance, it is critical to use the proper colors for a dark or light background, as shown.

CMYK-Color Brand Identity

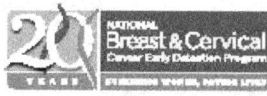

C0 M22 Y0 K0 · C0 M95 Y0 K25 · C80 M0 Y30 K10

1-Color Brand Identity (black)

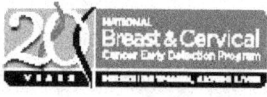

30% · 60% · 100%

NBCCEDP BACKGROUND COLOR USE

Use the CMYK-color or 1-color (black) version of the NBCCEDP 20th Anniversary Brand Identity when applying it to a white or light/mid-tone background. (See examples below)

Use the CMYK-color or 1-color (black) version with white rule outline of the NBCCEDP 20th Anniversary Brand Identity when applying it to a mid/dark-tone or dark background. (See examples below)

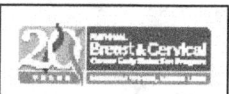 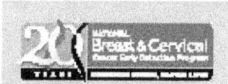 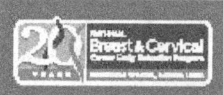 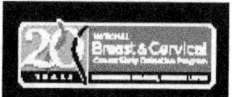

White Background · Light/Mid-tone Background · Mid/Dark-tone Background · Dark Background

SIZING AND POSITIONING

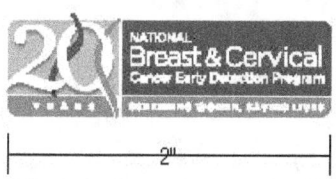

2"

Brand identity should never be smaller than 2" wide.

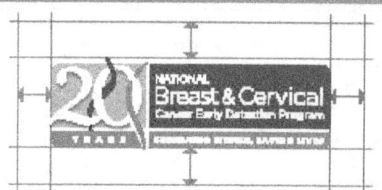

Leave clear space approximately 1/4" on all sides of the brand identity.

PROHIBITED USES

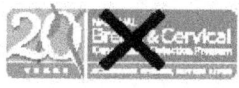 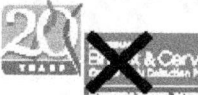 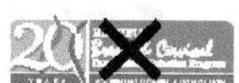 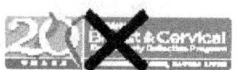

Do not alter the color of the brand identity.

Do not alter the position of the brand identity.

Do not alter or substitute the Wordmark or Tagline font from its existing form.

Brand identity must be re-sized in correct proportion.

National Breast and Cervical Cancer Early Detection Program
Affiliating with the National Program

The NBCCEDP or 20th Anniversary Brand Identity can be placed above or next to your program logo to show your affiliation with the national program. A text badge may also be used in conjunction with your logo.

SIZING AND POSITIONING — NBCCEDP AND 20TH ANNIVERSARY BRAND IDENTITIES

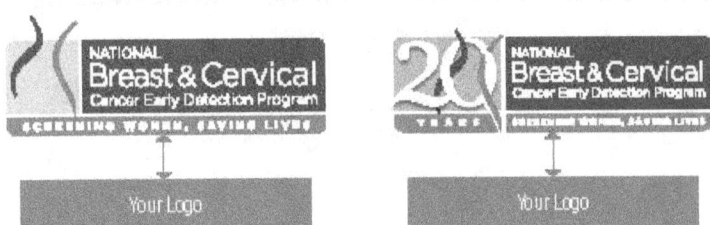

Stacked version of the combined branding elements should never be smaller than 2" wide. Leave a minimum of 1/4" clear space between the NBCCEDP Brand Identity or the 20th Anniversary Brand Identity and Your Logo. We recommend that the NBCCEDP Brand Identity and the 20th Anniversary Brand Identity be placed ABOVE Your Logo.

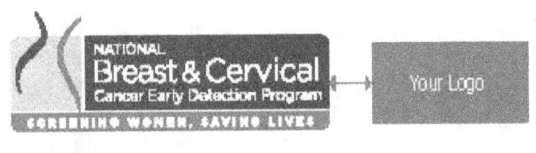

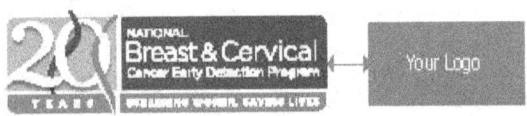

Side by side version of the combined branding elements should never be smaller than 5/8" high. Leave a minimum of 1/4" clear space between the NBCCEDP Brand Identity or the 20th Anniversary Brand Identity and Your Logo. We recommend that the NBCCEDP Brand Identity and the 20th Anniversary Brand Identity be placed to the LEFT of Your Logo.

PROHIBITED USES

Do not place Your Logo above the NBCCEDP Brand Identity or the 20th Anniversary Brand Identity.

Do not place Your Logo to the left of the NBCCEDP Brand Identity or the 20th Anniversary Brand Identity.

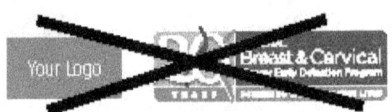

The NBCCEDP Text Badge provides programs with another opportunity to affiliate with CDC and NBCCEDP. The text badge can be placed next to or below your logo on your materials to show your affiliation with the national program.

NBCCEDP TEXT BADGE

In Partnership with CDC's National Breast and Cervical Cancer Early Detection Program

Horizontal Text Badge

In Partnership with CDC's National Breast and Cervical Cancer Early Detection Program

Vertical Text Badge

Text badge font: Gotham Book Italic

The Text Badge should only be printed as black (on light background) or white (on dark background).

SIZING AND POSITIONING — NBCCEDP TEXT BADGE

In Partnership with CDC's National Breast and Cervical Cancer Early Detection Program

2.5"

Horizontal Text Badge should never be smaller than 2.5" wide.

In Partnership with CDC's National Breast and Cervical Cancer Early Detection Program

1.5"

Vertical Text Badge should never be smaller than 1.5" wide.

Leave a minimum of 1/8" **clear space** between the Text Badge and Your Logo.

The Horizontal Text Badge is ALWAYS placed BELOW Your Logo.

The Vertical Text Badge is ALWAYS placed to the RIGHT of Your Logo.

Your Logo

In Partnership with CDC's National Breast and Cervical Cancer Early Detection Program

Your Logo | *In Partnership with CDC's National Breast and Cervical Cancer Early Detection Program*

PROHIBITED USES

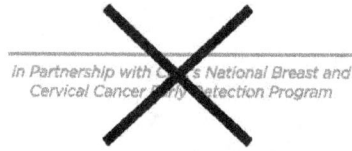

In Partnership with CDC's National Breast and Cervical Cancer Early Detection Program

Do not alter the color of the Text Badge.

In Partnership with CDC's National Breast and Cervical Cancer Early Detection Program

Do not alter or substitute the font of the Text Badge.

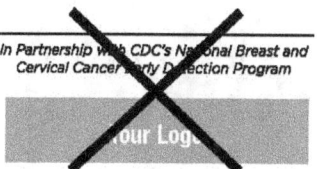

In Partnership with CDC's National Breast and Cervical Cancer Early Detection Program

Your Logo

Do not alter the position of the Text Badge.

National Breast and Cervical Cancer Early Detection Program Brand Identity Agreement Form

I have read and understand the *National Breast and Cervical Cancer Early Detection Program (NBCCEDP) Brand Identity Usage Terms and Conditions*. I agree to follow these Terms and Conditions and will only use the brand identities provided by the CDC for activity(ies) and dates indicated below on this form. To use the brand identities for additional purposes/activities or dates, I will submit another "Brand Identity Agreement" form. I recognize that by signing below, I am responsible for safeguarding the use of the brand identities and will not allow them to be used by others, especially by companies or individuals who sell products and/or services. I understand that the CDC, at its sole discretion, may disapprove or rescind its approval of any use that fails to comply with these Terms and Conditions. CDC approval of a request to use the NBCCEDP brand identity and tagline does not constitute endorsement of any private product or service, and does not create any right, benefit, or interest against the United States.

Your Name/Title:

Organization:

Address:

Web Site (if applicable):

E-Mail Address:

Phone Number:

Description of Request to Use NBCCEDP Brand Identities: *Please indicate what items will include the NBCCEDP or 20th Anniversary Brand Identities, intended target audience(s), what other logos will appear with the NBCCEDP brand identity, and additional relevant information.*

Signature:

Please return this form to the CDC prior to using the NBCCEDP brand identities on your program's materials: Melonie Thomas via e-mail at mqt8@cdc.gov or fax to (770) 488-3230. Should there be any questions or clarification needs regarding your indicated use of the brand identities, the CDC will contact you directly.